Advances in Hyperspectral and Multispectral Optical Spectroscopy and Imaging of Tissue

Advances in Hyperspectral and Multispectral Optical Spectroscopy and Imaging of Tissue

Editors

Vladislav Toronov
Mamadou Diop
Angelo Sassaroli
Ilias Tachtsidis

MDPI • Basel • Beijing • Wuhan • Barcelona • Belgrade • Manchester • Tokyo • Cluj • Tianjin

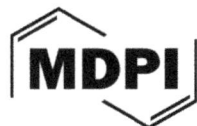

Editors
Vladislav Toronov
Toronto Metropolitan University
Canada

Mamadou Diop
Western University
Canada

Angelo Sassaroli
Tufts University
USA

Ilias Tachtsidis
University College London
UK

Editorial Office
MDPI
St. Alban-Anlage 66
4052 Basel, Switzerland

This is a reprint of articles from the Special Issue published online in the open access journal *Applied Sciences* (ISSN 2076-3417) (available at: https://www.mdpi.com/journal/applsci/special_issues/tissue_optical_Imaging).

For citation purposes, cite each article independently as indicated on the article page online and as indicated below:

LastName, A.A.; LastName, B.B.; LastName, C.C. Article Title. *Journal Name* **Year**, *Volume Number*, Page Range.

ISBN 978-3-0365-4477-9 (Hbk)
ISBN 978-3-0365-4478-6 (PDF)

© 2022 by the authors. Articles in this book are Open Access and distributed under the Creative Commons Attribution (CC BY) license, which allows users to download, copy and build upon published articles, as long as the author and publisher are properly credited, which ensures maximum dissemination and a wider impact of our publications.

The book as a whole is distributed by MDPI under the terms and conditions of the Creative Commons license CC BY-NC-ND.

Contents

Vladislav Toronov
Advances in Hyperspectral and Multispectral Optical Spectroscopy and Imaging of Tissue
Reprinted from: *Appl. Sci.* **2022**, *12*, 3543, doi:10.3390/app12073543 1

Frédéric Lange, Luca Giannoni and Ilias Tachtsidis
The Use of Supercontinuum Laser Sources in Biomedical Diffuse Optics: Unlocking the Power of Multispectral Imaging
Reprinted from: *Appl. Sci.* **2021**, *11*, 4616, doi:10.3390/app11104616 3

Zahida Guerouah, Steve Lin and Vladislav Toronov
Measurement of Adult Human Brain Responses to Breath-Holding by Multi-Distance Hyperspectral Near-Infrared Spectroscopy
Reprinted from: *Appl. Sci.* **2022**, *12*, 371, doi:10.3390/app12010371 35

Giles Blaney, Ryan Donaldson, Samee Mushtak, Han Nguyen, Lydia Vignale, Cristianne Fernandez, Thao Pham, Angelo Sassaroli and Sergio Fantini
Dual-Slope Diffuse Reflectance Instrument for Calibration-Free Broadband Spectroscopy
Reprinted from: *Appl. Sci.* **2021**, *11*, 1757, doi:10.3390/app11041757 51

Maxime D. Slooter, Sanne M. A. Jansen, Paul R. Bloemen, Richard M. van den Elzen, Leah S. Wilk, Ton G. van Leeuwen, Mark I. van Berge Henegouwen, Daniel M. de Bruin and Suzanne S. Gisbertz
Comparison of Optical Imaging Techniques to Quantitatively Assess the Perfusion of the Gastric Conduit during Oesophagectomy
Reprinted from: *Appl. Sci.* **2020**, *10*, 5522, doi:10.3390/app10165522 65

Charly Caredda, Laurent Mahieu-Williame, Raphaël Sablong, Michaël Sdika, Jacques Guyotat and Bruno Montcel
Optimal Spectral Combination of a Hyperspectral Camera for Intraoperative Hemodynamic and Metabolic Brain Mapping
Reprinted from: *Appl. Sci.* **2020**, *10*, 5158, doi:10.3390/app10155158 77

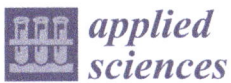

Editorial

Advances in Hyperspectral and Multispectral Optical Spectroscopy and Imaging of Tissue

Vladislav Toronov [1,2]

1 Department of Physics, Faculty of Science, Ryerson University, 350 Victoria Street, Toronto, ON M5B 2K3, Canada; toronov@ryerson.ca
2 Institute of Biomedical Engineering, Science and Technology (iBEST), Li Ka-Shing Knowledge Institute, 7th Floor, LKS 735, 209 Victoria Street, Toronto, ON M5B 1T8, Canada

Citation: Toronov, V. Advances in Hyperspectral and Multispectral Optical Spectroscopy and Imaging of Tissue. *Appl. Sci.* 2022, 12, 3543. https://doi.org/10.3390/app12073543

Received: 21 March 2022
Accepted: 29 March 2022
Published: 31 March 2022

Publisher's Note: MDPI stays neutral with regard to jurisdictional claims in published maps and institutional affiliations.

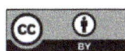

Copyright: © 2022 by the author. Licensee MDPI, Basel, Switzerland. This article is an open access article distributed under the terms and conditions of the Creative Commons Attribution (CC BY) license (https:// creativecommons.org/licenses/by/ 4.0/).

1. Introduction

Optical imaging and characterization of tissue has become a huge applied field due to the advantages of the optical analysis methods, which include non-invasiveness, portability, high sensitivity, and high spectral specificity. This research field continues to grow and spread in many different directions due to the development of new light sources and detectors, such as, for example, the supercontinuum and tunable lasers, portable highly sensitive spectrometers, multiwavelength photoacoustic imagers, due to novel methods of data analysis, such as the machine-learning methods of spectral analysis, and due to novel applications, such as the imaging of embryogenesis or monitoring of the cerebral oxygen metabolism. Polarization analysis of the anisotropy of optical, mechanical, and electrical properties of materials is another active research direction in hyperspectral imaging from THz to IR spectral ranges.

The purpose of this Special Issue is to provide an overview of recent advances in the methods of tissue imaging and characterization, which benefit from using large numbers of optical wavelengths.

2. Review of Issue Contents

The human brain is an enchanting object of studies by near-infrared spectroscopy and imaging. In this Special Issue, Guerouah et al. [1] has contributed a profound study of the responses of adult human brain to breath-holding challenges by the hyperspectral near-infrared spectroscopy (hNIRS). This work examined brain signals across the entire near-infrared therapeutic spectral window and showed the critical role of the short-distance channel for the robust measurements of the hemodynamic and metabolic changes in the brain.

Hyperspectral spectroscopy and imaging requires broadband light sources. In the last 20 years, supercontinuum laser sources covering wide spectral bandwidths at high spectral power and fast switching have been developed. Lange et al. [2] contributed a timely and comprehensive review of the features and biomedical and clinical applications of supercontinuum laser sources.

Near-infrared spectroscopy is a quantitative tool that allows for the inspection and characterization of biological tissues and other turbid media such as wood, food and pharmaceutical products, soil, marble, etc. The quantitative accuracy of the medium characterization can be improved using hNIRS. In this Special Issue, Blaney et al. [3] reported a development of a calibration-free hNIRS system that can measure the absolute and broadband absorption and scattering spectra of turbid media.

The ability of the optical imaging techniques to provide real-time quantitative assessment of the biological tissue urges research on their use for tissue monitoring during surgeries. Slooter et al. [4] studied the utility of the measuring multiple tissue parameters simultaneously by four optical techniques operating at different wavelengths of light: optical coherence tomography (1300 nm), sidestream darkfield microscopy (530 nm), laser speckle contrast imaging (785 nm), and fluorescence angiography (~800 nm) of the gastric conduit during esophagectomy.

Neurosurgical procedures on the open human brain require localization of the functional cortical areas in real time. A Monte Carlo simulation study by Caredda et al. [5] showed feasibility to accurately quantify the oxy- and deoxy-hemoglobin and cytochrome-c-oxidase responses to neuronal activation and to obtain the spatial maps of these responses using a setup consisting of a while light source and a hyperspectral or a standard RGB camera.

3. Conclusions

This Special Issue is of interest for the developers and potential users of clinical brain and tissue optical monitors, and for the researchers studying brain physiology and functional brain activity.

Funding: This research received no external funding.

Conflicts of Interest: The author declares no conflict of interest.

References

1. Guerouah, Z.; Lin, S.; Toronov, V. Measurement of Adult Human Brain Responses to Breath-Holding by Multi-Distance Hyperspectral Near-Infrared Spectroscopy. *Appl. Sci.* **2022**, *12*, 371. [CrossRef]
2. Lange, F.; Giannoni, L.; Tachtsidis, I. The Use of Supercontinuum Laser Sources in Biomedical Diffuse Optics: Unlocking the Power of Multispectral Imaging. *Appl. Sci.* **2021**, *11*, 4616. [CrossRef]
3. Blaney, G.; Donaldson, R.; Mushtak, S.; Nguyen, H.; Vignale, L.; Fernandez, C.; Pham, T.; Sassaroli, A.; Fantini, S. Dual-Slope Diffuse Reflectance Instrument for Calibration-Free Broadband Spectroscopy. *Appl. Sci.* **2021**, *11*, 1757. [CrossRef]
4. Slooter, M.; Jansen, S.; Bloemen, P.; van den Elzen, R.; Wilk, L.; van Leeuwen, T.; van Berge Henegouwen, M.; de Bruin, D.; Gisbertz, S. Comparison of Optical Imaging Techniques to Quantitatively Assess the Perfusion of the Gastric Conduit during Oesophagectomy. *Appl. Sci.* **2020**, *10*, 5522. [CrossRef]
5. Caredda, C.; Mahieu-Williame, L.; Sablong, R.; Sdika, M.; Guyotat, J.; Montcel, B. Optimal Spectral Combination of a Hyperspectral Camera for Intraoperative Hemodynamic and Metabolic Brain Mapping. *Appl. Sci.* **2020**, *10*, 5158. [CrossRef]

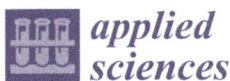

Review

The Use of Supercontinuum Laser Sources in Biomedical Diffuse Optics: Unlocking the Power of Multispectral Imaging

Frédéric Lange [1,*], Luca Giannoni [1,2,3] and Ilias Tachtsidis [1]

1. Biomedical Optics Research Laboratory, Department of Medical Physics and Biomedical Engineering, University College London, London WC1E 6BT, UK; giannoni@lens.unifi.it (L.G.); i.tachtsidis@ucl.ac.uk (I.T.)
2. National Institute of Optics, National Research Council, 50019 Sesto Fiorentino, Italy
3. European Laboratory for Non-linear Spectroscopy, 50019 Sesto Fiorentino, Italy
* Correspondence: f.lange@ucl.ac.uk

Abstract: Optical techniques based on diffuse optics have been around for decades now and are making their way into the day-to-day medical applications. Even though the physics foundations of these techniques have been known for many years, practical implementation of these technique were hindered by technological limitations, mainly from the light sources and/or detection electronics. In the past 20 years, the developments of supercontinuum laser (SCL) enabled to unlock some of these limitations, enabling the development of system and methodologies relevant for medical use, notably in terms of spectral monitoring. In this review, we focus on the use of SCL in biomedical diffuse optics, from instrumentation and methods developments to their use for medical applications. A total of 95 publications were identified, from 1993 to 2021. We discuss the advantages of the SCL to cover a large spectral bandwidth with a high spectral power and fast switching against the disadvantages of cost, bulkiness, and long warm up times. Finally, we summarize the utility of using such light sources in the development and application of diffuse optics in biomedical sciences and clinical applications.

Keywords: supercontinuum laser; NIRS; tissue optics; diffuse optics

1. Introduction

Non-invasive optical monitoring of the human physiology has been a great asset in the medical diagnosis over the last decades [1], and this field is still expanding as technological advances drives the development of new instruments for use in various medical applications [2]. One of the main techniques of optical monitoring of biological tissues is near-infrared spectroscopy (NIRS). It is based on the use of light between 650 and 900 nm, which is within the so-called "transparency window". Within this light window, the optical absorption of biological tissue is at its lowest and light scattering is sufficiently high so the propagation of light in tissue is facilitated. Therefore, NIRS provides a way to gather information from deep into the tissue [3]. As one of the main absorbers in this window is the hemoglobin, in its oxygenated and deoxygenated forms (oxy- and deoxy-hemoglobin ([HbO_2] and [HHb], respectively), NIRS has been broadly used to quantify the changes in oxygenation of various tissues like muscle and brain [4]. This ability to quantify oxygenation non-invasively, and in real time has helped NIRS to become a standard technique in the labs. However, a few pitfalls are still holding back its wide adoption at a clinical level. Indeed, most of the widespread techniques used for NIRS are based on the so-called continuous wave (CW) technique where the tissue is illuminated with a non-coherent light and the variation in light intensity is collected at the detector [5]. In this configuration, it is harder to estimate absolute quantities, as the underlying optical properties of the tissue (mainly absorption and scattering coefficient) cannot be measured, and the scattering properties are assumed to be fixed (i.e., in time and for every subject). Therefore, most of the CW-NIRS systems only quantify the changes in hemoglobin concentration. This can be a drawback for clinical use, as an absolute comparison between two patients cannot be done unless you involve a well-controlled physiological stimulus. The other drawback is that the measurement is often performed with only two wavelengths, the minimum necessary to retrieve two absorbing compounds [HbO$_2$] and [HHb]. However, the contribution of other chromophores is either neglected (like collagen), or assumed and fixed, like water. This results in an increase in the physiological noise, which reduces the accuracy of the measurement.

These drawbacks have been tackled over the recent years, and some new techniques and instrumentation enabled researchers to work around these drawbacks. Firstly, one can use more advanced CW-NIRS techniques in order to extract absolute information about the tissue. We can cite the broadband NIRS that also has the capability to extract absolute information of tissue optical properties [6]. The added benefits of this technique are that, as it uses a large number of wavelength (typically more than a hundred), it can perform a true spectroscopic analysis, hence also gathering information about other chromophores like cytochromes, water, and fat [6]. This extra information enables having a complete optical view of the tissue under investigations. Moreover, on top of providing a more precise view of the oxygenation, the use of many wavelengths enables targeting novel optical contrasts, like the oxidative state of the cytochrome-c-oxidase (oxCCO) which is a biomarker of metabolism [7].

However, even though these improvements are promising, performing a true spectroscopic measurement on tissue using NIRS is still challenging. One of the main issues is the penetration depth of the light and the contamination of the tissues of interest by the upper layers (i.e., skin) [3]. Indeed, the tissues are often modelled as homogeneous for simplicity, even though this hypothesis is not true. Therefore, new methodologies are required to enhance the discrimination between different tissue types, thus improving the accuracy of the measurement.

It is well known that the time-domain NIRS (TD-NIRS) is the most advanced and accurate type of measurement, capable of retrieving absolute information and to discriminate between shallow and deep tissue [8]. Briefly, in TD-NIRS an ultra-short light impulse (typically in the picosecond range) illuminates the tissue. Tissue has the effect of attenuating and broadening the re-emitted pulse (the resulting pulse-width is typically few nanoseconds wide). The measured signal is typically called a temporal point spread function (TPSF) or distribution of time of flights (DTOFs) of photons. Indeed, what is measured here is the histogram of the arrival time of photons. Thus, the amount of information acquired by TD-NIRS systems outstrips the classical CW-NIRS, which only acquires the intensity. From these DTOF, various data processing methods can be employed to extract information about the tissue. It is out of the scope of this paper to detail these methods, but the interested reader can refer to the following reviews for a more in-depth description of TD-NIRS methodologies [9,10], and for a special focus on broadband TD-NIRS [11], which will be largely discussed in the present work.

The extraction of more accurate information with TD-NIRS comes at the cost of a more complex instrumentation, requiring pulsed-laser source (pulse in order of MHz) and fast electronic and sensitive detectors in order to be able to unlock single photon counting. Thus, even though TD-NIRS has been around for many decades now and has been developed in parallel to CW-NIRS, these more specific requirements have hindered its development. Nevertheless, much progress has been made over the last two decades, and TD-NIRS is closing the gap with CW-NIRS in terms of user's adoption.

One of the key developments that has promoted the development of TD-NIRS is the supercontinuum laser (SCL) sources, which provide a white laser source, with a high power (several watts) and a very short pulse width (typical less than 10 ps) at several tens of MHz. Indeed, these characteristics are essential in order to develop reliable TD-NIRS systems, that started to be developed in the nineties. During these early days of development, no commercial pulsed laser diodes were available, and one had to rely on homemade SC generation or Ti-Sapphire lasers in order to be able to produce a coherence pulsed light with a spectral power density sufficient to be detected by the photon counting electronic.

Therefore, SCL sources have been a true driver of TD-NIRS development in the early days, and have more recently unlocked new horizons like spectroscopy, which have broadened the fields of applications.

Finally, besides traditional sparse measurement of tissue properties with diffuse optics, Diffuse Optical Tomography (DOT) has also been rapidly expending in the past decades. This imaging technique is based on the acquisition of a large number of channels, coupled to a more refined data analysis, based on anatomically realistic models of tissue. This allows to reconstruct 3D spatial distribution of optical/physiological parameters of the tissues, rather than providing tissue information on a limited number of points. An extension of this technique is called fluorescence DOT, that uses extrinsic near-infrared fluorescent dyes which targets specific tissues to harvest extra information and enable molecular imaging. The interested reader can refer to reviews [12,13] for more information about these techniques. We will see that SCL sources have also a role to play in order to improve the performances of the DOT instruments.

In this work, we will review the use of SCL in the field of biomedical diffuse optics. Thus, we will begin by a short overview of the history and basic principle of supercontinuum generation. Then, we will review works that have been using SCL in biomedical diffuse optics, from the instrument development to the application. Finally, we will summarize and highlight the strength and weakness of SCL for these applications and show what areas can benefits from its use.

2. History and Basic Principles of Supercontinuum Lasers

Supercontinuum (SC) lasers are broadband, coherent light sources that are capable of combining the wide spectral range of conventional white lamps (including UV, visible and IR light) with the optical performances of single-mode lasers, in particular their high output intensity, the capability of fast, pulsed emission, and the fine collimation of the beam down to diffraction limit. Such characteristics make this type of photonic technology highly versatile for a number of applications, in particular in biomedical optics and biophotonics, thanks also to recent advancement towards making SC lasers more compact and affordable [14].

The physical process of optical SC generation was discovered and studied in the 60 s and 70 s with milestones publications by Alfano and Shapiro [15,16]. It is based on the propagation of extreme non-linear effects from a narrow-bandwidth pulsed laser beam in order to generate a broadening of the overall spectrum of the emitted light. These non-linear effects typically include self-phase modulation, four-wave mixing, Raman scattering, and solitons dynamics, among others [14,17]. The propagation of these effects is performed by dispersing the pulsed laser beam through a non-linear material. These can range from bulk materials, such as simple water cells, silicas, or gases (as in the earliest attempts of SC generation), to more advanced crystal-structured optical fibres [17,18].

Early SC lasers using bulk materials for non-linear propagation were limited in the efficiency of coupling the input laser light with these propagating material (coupling efficiencies stood at below 10%) and thus they were able to only achieve ranges of about 200–300 nm, with pulses duration in the order of tens of nanoseconds. Further developments in SC generation efficiency and coupling using optic fibres lead to enlarging the range up to 1–2 μm and increasing the pulse duration to the range of picoseconds (for commercial, compact lasers), or even femtoseconds (for research-grade, benchtop lasers) [18]. A critical turning point for modern SC lasers to achieve such high performances was the invention and application of photonic crystal fibres (PCF), a particular type of microstructured optic fibre (Figure 1).

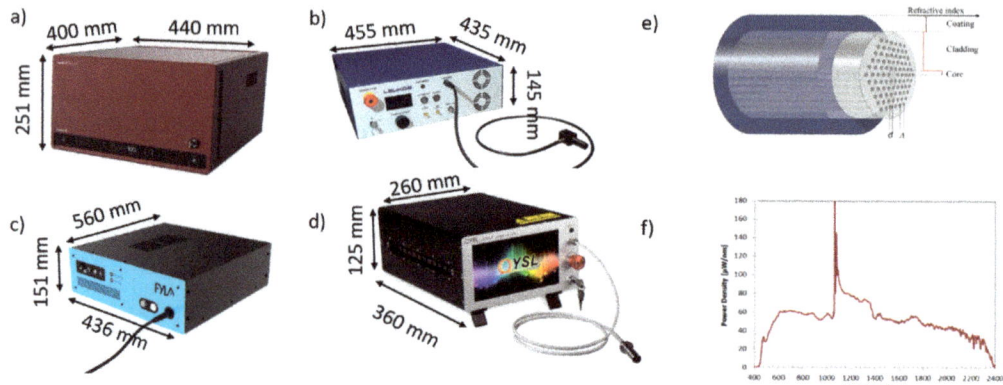

Figure 1. Example of commercial SC laser sources and their typical spectra. (**a**) Fianium source, (**b**) Leukos source, (**c**) FYLA source, (**d**) YSL source. (**e**) Schematic of the classical triangular cladding single-core photonic crystal fiber in which light is guided in a solid core embedded in a triangular lattice of air holes. The fiber structure is determined by the hole-size, d, and the hole-pitch, Λ. Like standard fibers, the PCF is coated with a high index polymer for protection and to strip off cladding-modes. Extracted from the application note on supercontinuum generation in photonic crystal fibers by NKT. (**f**) Example of full spectrum generated by a SC laser, showing the width of the broadband emission and the central peak wavelength that is a residual of the single-mode laser used for SC generation. The spectrum is taken from the SuperK COMPACT SC laser manufactured by NKT Photonics (https://www.nktphotonics.com/lasers-fibers/product/superk-compact-supercontinuum-lasers/, accessed date: 1 November 2021).

PCFs, invented in 1996 [19], are currently the most used non-linear propagating materials for SC generation [17,18]. As the name suggests, this class of optic fibres is based on recreating the optical properties of crystalline structures, in particular their photonic bandgap effect, by combining various high and low refractive indexes in their inner structure. Such features can be achieved in different manners, which typically define the given category of PCFs [20]: (1) hollow-core PCFs present a central hole in their structures, filled with air; (2) holey PCFs are composed of a matrix of several air-filled holes in their cross-sections that is interspersed with the core material; (3) solid-core PCFs involves a solid core surrounded by a matrix of air-filled holes.

PCFs offer high coupling efficiencies and low power losses, thus allowing ultra-broadband, high-brightness SC generation at cost-effective access [17,21]. SC lasers based on PCFs used in biomedical optics applications can typically generate broad spectrum spanning from 350 to 2400 nm, generally showing a central sharp peak which is a residual of the original shape of the pulsed beam. An example of this is shown in Figure 1. Most commercial SC lasers show performances similar to pulsed laser diodes, with integrated output power up to tens of watts and the capability of generating pulses in the order of picoseconds and repetition rates of tens of MHz [22].

Finally, we can report that in the recent year, more companies are able to provide ready-to-use SC solution. A search from the website https://www.rp-photonics.com (accessed date: 1 November 2021), displays at least 4 companies manufacturing SCL: NKT photonics, who recently acquired the former UK company Fianium (www.nktphotonics.com, accessed date: 1 November 2021), LEUKOS (www.leukos-systems.com, accessed date: 1 November 2021), FYLA (www.fyla.com, accessed date: 1 November 2021) and YSL photonics (www.yslphotonics.com, accessed date: 1 November 2021). Figure 1 displays pictures of different SCL offered by these companies.

3. The Use of Supercontinuum Lasers in Biomedical Diffuse Optics

The focus of the present review was to evaluate the use of SCL in biomedical diffuse optics, from the systems and methodological developments to their medical applications.

Therefore, papers were identified using PubMed, Scopus, and Web of Science, searching for a combination of keywords including (supercontinuum laser | white laser) and (diffuse optics | NIRS). Moreover, a manual search from articles' references was performed and the personal reference library of the authors of the current papers has also been searched. Papers were rejected if no SCL was used in the method section of the reported work, if the application was not medically related, if they were reviews or if the method was not purely optical (i.e., no photoacoustic papers). A total of 95 publications covering a variety of focus were identified. We have identified 4 main categories of publications: system development (31 studies), optical properties estimation (16 studies), methodology (43 studies) and application (5 studies). Table 1 provides a summary of the main characteristics of the SCL used in the studies reported in this review, Figure 2 shows pictures of the instrumentation typically used, and Figure 3 presents typical output in terms of datatypes of such systems. Moreover, a summary of the studies included in this review is presented in Table 2 and includes the system used, the year, the category of the study and the target of the study. Finally, Figure 4 summarizes the main topics and characteristic of the systems used in the reviewed publications and shows the number of publications over the last 30 years that report the use of SCL in biomedical diffuse optics.

3.1. Novel Instrument Developement

The first paper reporting the use of a supercontinuum laser in biomedical diffuse optics was reported in the early nineties [29–31] by a group based at the Lund Laser Centre (LLC, Lund, Sweden). The femtosecond white light supercontinuum was generated by a Terawatt laser running at 10 Hz. The spectral decomposition was performed on the detection side, by coupling an imaging spectrometer and a streak camera, enabling to acquire parallelly the DTOF at all wavelengths. To improve the signal-to-noise ratio, the measurement had to be repeated for several laser shots, but the overall acquisition time was of just a few minutes, which is acceptable when no dynamic contrast is targeted. Using such a system, the very first in vivo absorption and scattering spectra of the female breast were acquired from 650 to 850 nm. This system was then updated in the early 2000s with a supercontinuum generation system based on a crystal fibre, which allowed to increase the optical power of the SCL generation [32].

Table 1. List of the SC laser-based systems used in the publications reviewed, with their principal characteristics. SC: SuperContinuum, FWHM: Full Widht at Half Maximum, CCD: Charge-Coupled Device, ICCD: Intensified Charge-Coupled Device, PMT: PhotoMultiplier Tube, SPAD: Single-Photon Avalanche Diode, SiPM: Silicon PhotoMultiplier, HPM: Hybrid Photodetector Module, sCMOS: scientific Complementary Metal–Oxide–Semiconductor, NIR: Near InfraRed.

System ID	Group	Year	SC Laser Type/Model	Spectral Capacity	Power (mW)	Repetition Rate (kHz)	Pulse Width (ps)	Detector Type	N° of Channels
				SC Laser System Characteristics				System Detection Characteristics	
1	Lund Institute of Technology, Lund, Sweden	1993	In-house	White light centred at 792 nm	1000	0.01	200	CCD camera	NA
2	Politecnico di Milano, Milan, Italy	2004	In-house	550–1100 nm	40	85,000	50–100	PMT	16
3	Lund Institute of Technology, Lund, Sweden	2004	In-house	500–1200 nm	NA	80,000	100	Streak camera	NA
4	Université Jean Monnet, Saint-Etienne, France.	2005	In-house	450–950 nm	1	1	170	Streak camera	NA
5	Politecnico di Milano, Milan, Italy	2006	In-house	550–1050 nm 120 bands	100	NA	60–140	PMT	32
6	Politecnico di Milano, Milan, Italy	2007	SC450, Fianium	(600–1000 nm) FWHM = 5–20 nm	2600 (total)	20,000	10	SPAD	1
7	Lund University, Lund, Sweden	2009	SC500, Fianium	650–1400 nm	NA	80,000	50	PMT	2
8	Northeastern University, Boston, United States	2010	Koheras SuperK, NKT Photonics	550–850 nm	NA	80,000	30	PMT	16
9	National Optics Institute, Québec, Canada	2010	SC400, Fianium	Filtered at 660 nm	NA	40,000	90	PMT	1
10	Physikalisch-Technische Bundesanstalt, Berlin, Germany	2011	Fianium (model NA)	Tuned at 690 nm	NA	20,000	100	SPAD	1
11	University of California, Irvine, United States	2012	SC450, Fianium	680–850 nm	2000	20,000	3	PMT	2
12	Institute of Biocybernetics and Biomedical Engineering Polish Academy of Sciences, Warsaw, Poland	2012	SC450-4 (Fianium)	685–860, 16 bands	NA	40,000	NA	PMT	16
13	Politecnico di Milano, Milan, Italy	2012	SC450, Fianium	1100–1700 nm FWHM = 6.6–20.7 nm	6000 (total)	40,000	10	SPAD	1
14	Massachusetts General Hospital, Boston, United States	2013	SC600-8, Fianium	680, 710, 747, 760, 800, 820, 830, 840 nm	9000 (total)	60,000	NA	ICCD	175
15	Politecnico di Milano, Milan, Italy	2010	SuperK Extreme, NKT Photonics	600–1100 m	5000 (total)	2000–80,000	10	PMT	1

Table 1. Cont.

System ID	Group	Year	SC Laser Type/Model	Spectral Capacity	Power (mW)	Repetition Rate (kHz)	Pulse Width (ps)	Detector Type	N° of Channels
16	Katholieke Universiteit Leuven, Leuven, Belgium	2012	SC450-4, Fianium	450–2400 nm	4000 (total)	NA	NA	PINdiode	1
17	University College London, London, United Kingdom	2014	SC450, Fianium	690, 750, 800, 850 nm	4.5	40,000	4	PMT	32
18	Politecnico di Milano, Milan, Italy	2014	SC500-6, Fianium	Tuned at 800 nm	NA	40,500	NA	HPM	1
19	CREATIS, Université de Lyon, Lyon, France	2015	WhiteLase Micro, Fianium	500–1000 nm	10	2000	NA	ICCD	8
20	Politecnico di Milano, Milan, Italy	2015	SC450, Fianium	620 nm (40-nm bandwidth)	NA	80,000	NA	SPAD	1
21	Politecnico di Milano, Milan, Italy	2015	SC450, Fianium	750 nm (5-nm bandwidth)	NA	40,000	NA	SPAD	1
22	Politecnico di Milano, Milan, Italy	2015	SC450, Fianium	690 nm	NA	40,000	NA	SiPM	1
23	The City College of New York, New York, United States	2015	STM-2000-IR, Leukos	400–2500 nm	0.5/1 nm	NA	NA	IR-CCD	1
24	Politecnico di Milano, Milan, Italy	2015	SC450, Fianium	600–1350 nm	NA	40,000	NA	SiPM and PMT	2
25	Politecnico di Milano, Milan, Italy	2016	SC500-6, Fianium	760, 860 nm	30	40,500	NA	SPAD	1
26	Physikalisch-Technische Bundesanstalt, Berlin, Germany	2016	SC500-6, Fianium	Tuned at 650 nm	NA	40,500	100	SPAD	1
27	Politecnico di Milano, Milan, Italy	2017	Fianium (model NA)	750, 800, 850 nm	NA	40,000	NA	SPAD	2
28	State Key Laboratory of Precision Measuring Technology and Instruments, Tianjin University, Tianjin, China	2018	SC46 (YSL photonics)	1100–1350 nm (12 bands)	8000 (Total)	10–80,000	NA	InGaAs photodiode	1
29	Rensselaer Polytechnique Institute, Troy, United States	2018	MaiTai, Spectra Physics (1) SC Pro, YSL Photonics (2)	(1) 690–1040 nm FWHM = 15 nm (2) 400–2200 nm	(1) NA (2) 4000 (total)	(1) 80,000 (2) 25,000	(1) 100 (2) 150–200	PMT and NIR camera	2

Table 1. Cont.

System ID	Group	Year	SC Laser Type/Model	SC Laser System Characteristics					System Detection Characteristics	
				Spectral Capacity	Power (mW)	Repetition Rate (kHz)	Pulse Width (ps)	Detector Type	N° of Channels
30	Institute of Biocybernetics and Biomedical Engineering Polish Academy of Sciences, Warsaw, Poland	2018	SC450-4, Fianium	650–850 nm, 16 bands of 12.5 nm	NA	40,000–80,000	NA	PMT	1
31	University of Pennsylvania, Philadelphia, United States	2018	SuperK Extreme, NKT Photonics	730, 750, 786, 810, 830, 850 nm	NA	78,000	5	PMT	2
32	Physikalisch-Technische Bundesanstalt, Berlin, Germany	2019	FIU-15 PP, NKT Photonics	NA	NA	NA	NA	SPAD and HPM	2
33	University of Science and Technology, Trondheim, Norway	2019	SuperK Compact, NKT Photonics (1) SCT 500, Fyla (2)	NA	NA	20 (1) 20,000 (2)	NA	InGaAs detector	2
34	University of California, Irvine, United States	2019	SC400-2, Fianium	1000 bands (580–950 nm) FWHM = 17.25 nm (mean)	2000 (total)	NA	NA	sCMOS camera	NA
35	University College London, London, United Kingdom	2019	SC480-6, Fianium	16 bands (650–1100 nm) FWHM = 2–3 nm	6000 (total)	60,000	4	PMT	4
36	Physikalisch-Technische Bundesanstalt, Berlin, Germany	2019	SC500-6, Fianium	Tuned at 800 nm	NA	40,500	NA	HPM	1
37	Institute of Biocybernetics and Biomedical Engineering Polish Academy of Sciences, Warsaw, Poland	2020	FIU-15 PP, NKT Photonics	Tuned at 760 nm	NA	39,000	NA	HPM	1
38	University College London, London, United Kingdom	2021	WhiteLase Micro, Fianium	600, 630, 665, 784, 800, 818, 835, 851, 868, 881, 894 nm (FWHM = 6–11 nm)	0.06–0.11	NA	NA	sCMOS camera	NA
39	Biomedical Optics Research Laboratory, University Hospital Zurich and University of Zurich, Switzerland	2020	SuperK ExtremeEXR-15 (NKT)	Tuned at 800 nm	6000 (total)	80,000	NA	SPAD camera	NA

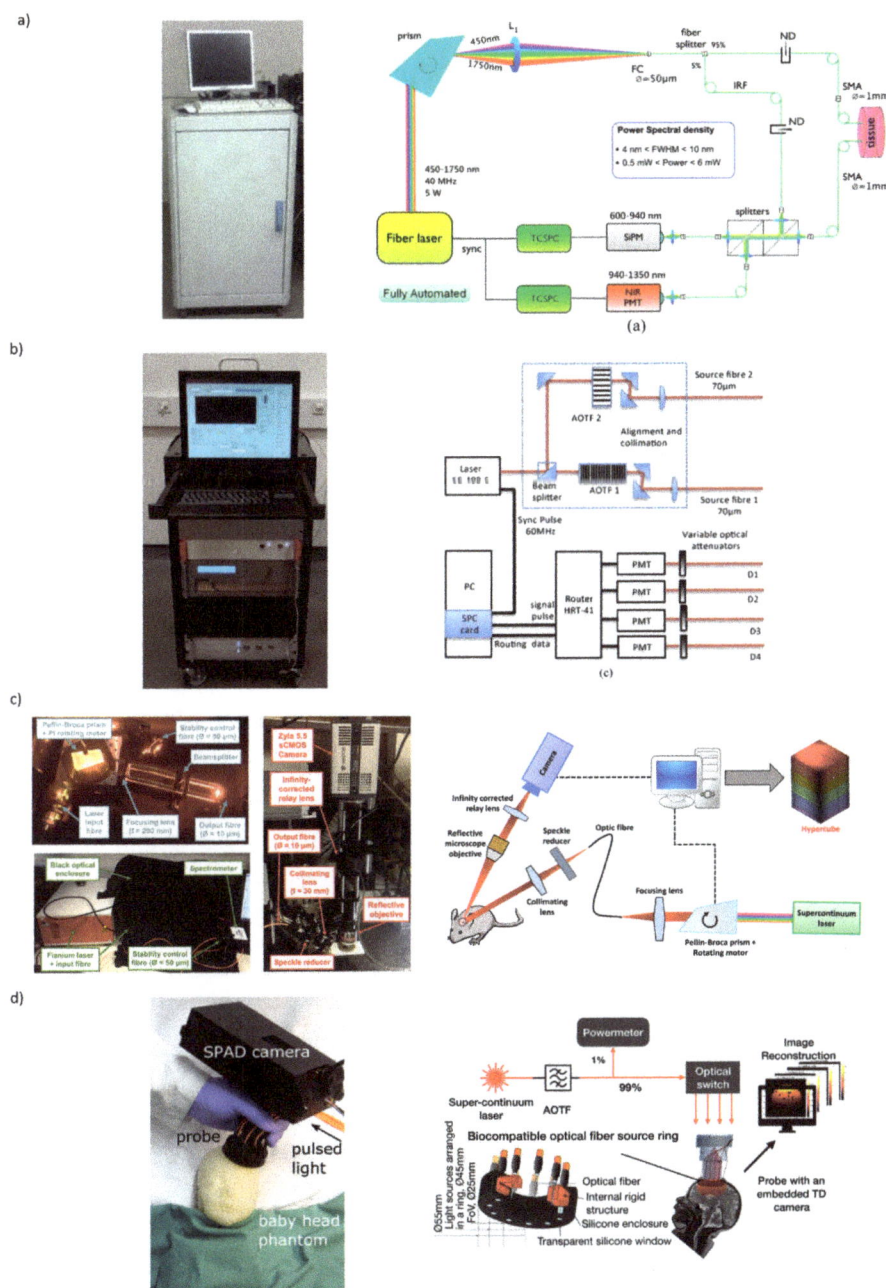

Figure 2. Pictures and schematic of various instruments based on SCL as a source. (**a**) TD-NIRS instrument aimed at broadband characterization of tissues. Figure reproduced from [23]. (**b**) TD-NIRS instrument aimed at monitoring both oxygenation and metabolism functional changes. Figure reproduced from [24]. (**c**) Preclinical instrument aimed at monitoring the exposed brain cortex of rodents. (reproduced with permission from [25], Copyright IEEE, 2021). (**d**) DOT system based on a SPAD camera aimed at functional brain monitoring in neonates. Figure reproduced from [26,27].

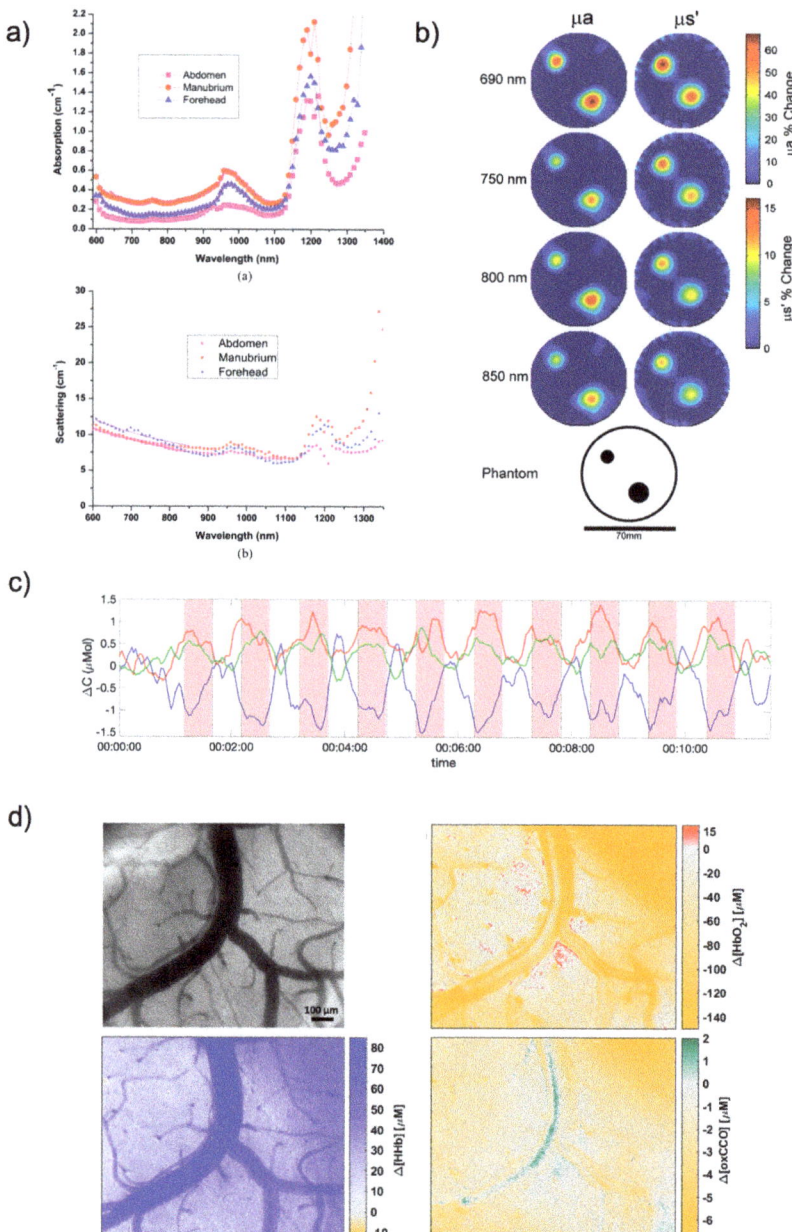

Figure 3. Example of typical data extracted form system based on SCL as sources. (**a**) absorption and reduce scattering coefficient of several tissues acquired the TD-NIRS system developed in ref [23]. Figure reproduced from [23]. (**b**) 2D maps of the changes in optical properties of a phantom using MONSTIR II. (reproduced with permission from [28], Copyright AIP Publishing, 2021). (**c**) Changes in [HbO2] (red), [HHb] (blue) and [oxCCO](green), in the occipital lobe, acquired with the MAESTROS system [24], during a typical brain activation. Data presented at the fNIRS conference in Tokyo in 2018. (**d**) Raw image and reconstructed variation in [HbO2], [HHb], and [oxCCO] acquired on the exposed cortex during anoxia. (reproduced with permission from [25], Copyright IEEE, 2021).

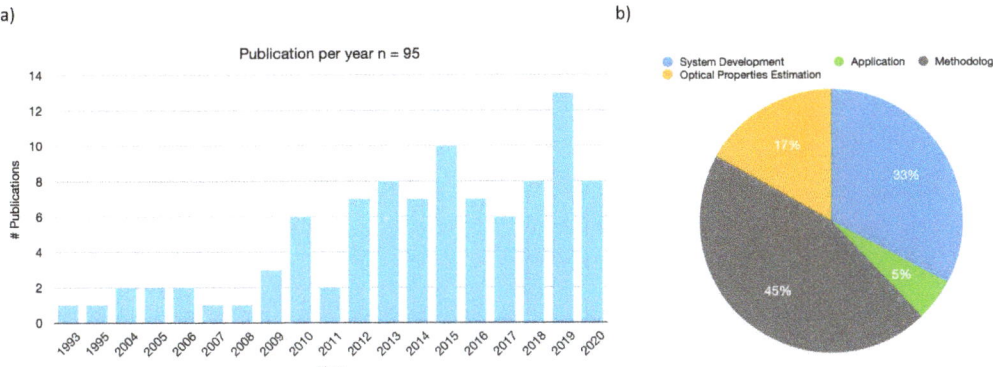

Figure 4. Summary of the literature review results. (**a**) Graph showing the number of publications using SCL in biomedical diffuse optics since the first study in 1993. (**b**) Summary of the main focus of the papers reviewed.

Parallel to these initial developments, a team based at Politecnico di Milano (POLIMI) produced a system able to characterise tissue between 610 and 1050 nm [33]. The system was however not based on a supercontinuum laser generation but on two tuneable lasers for the source, and the detection scheme was based on time-correlated single-photon counting (TCSPC), enabling light detection down to the single photon, which drastically improves the sensitivity of the system. This increased sensitivity is of great advantage to reduce the acquisition time and improve the light collection in the region where water absorption is high (900–1050). However, handling two lasers drastically increases the complexity and bulkiness of the system. Nevertheless, with that system, that team was able to record the optical properties of absorption and scattering of various tissues in-vivo [34–37]. The availability of commercial SCL sources gave rise to a new version of that system, where the 2 lasers were replaced by a SCL source coupled with a prism for the spectral selection [38]. This new source allowed to make the system more compact and transportable making it more suitable for the clinic. Moreover, the detector was also replaced (previously photomultiplier (PMT)) by a Single-Photon Avalanche Diode (SPAD) which enable to increase the spectral coverage, allowing a measurement between 600 and 1000 nm. This system could be used to characterise the optical and physiological properties of the tissue of the female breast. Another version of that system was developed, combining the SCL with a Ti-Sapphire laser to expand the spectral coverage to 1100 nm [39]. The SCL was used to cover the 600–900 nm and the Ti-Sapphire was used between 900 and 1100 nm. Indeed, even though the SCL could cover the entire considered wavelength band, the spectral resolution provided by the couple SCL/dispersion prism was too low to provide accurate results, as the source bandwidth increased with wavelength from 3 nm at 600 nm to 10 nm at 900 nm, and to approximately 15 nm at 1100 nm with that solution. This instrument has indeed been used to demonstrate that the broadening of the spectral bandwidth effect could impair the results, as the spectral region within the bandpass that exhibits the lowest absorption will dominate, leading to significant underestimations of the absorption and distortions in the spectral shape [40]. The spectral quality of the acquired data being extremely important, having the narrowest bandwidth is a great advantage. To do so, using a SCL is thus a true advantage as it provides a high power across the entire spectra. However, the method used to filter the white light is very important. As it has been seen above, several techniques can be used, either filtering on the detection side with a spectrometer, or on the source side with a dispersive prism or using an acousto-optic tuneable filter (AOTF), as we will see in systems described below. The POLIMI team has compared the wavelength selection from a SCL with an AOTF and a prism. They have shown that one had to be careful when using AOTF, as they can produce side lobes in the selected bandpass, which can drastically impair the retrieval of the optical properties [41].

Nevertheless, the extension of the spectral coverage offered by this newly developed system was of particular interest, as several components, like lipid and collagen, have a distinct signature above 1000 nm. The LLC group also reported a similar system, based on a commercial SCL coupled with 2 AOTF and a detection scheme based on TCSPC with a coverage between 650 and 1400 nm [42]. The POLIMI group has then extended this work by focusing on the spectral window between 900 and 1700 nm, by using an InGaAs/InP SPAD as a detector [43–45]. Finally, they have produced a system able to cover the entire bandwidth from 600 to 1350 nm using a single SCL coupled with a prism for the wavelength selection, and 2 TCSPC cards couples with 2 detectors covering different bandwidth [23]. They managed to fix the issue of the spectral broadening induced by the prism by refining the optical chain. Additionally, this system was mounted on a 19-inch medical cart, making it easily used in a clinical environment. This system can be seen in Figure 2 and in an example of data in Figure 3. Moreover, by adjusting the detector used, the same instrument can be used to cover an even larger bandwidth, between 500 to 1700 nm [46].

With all these developments, POLIMI has been a major contributor to multispectral TD-NIRS and were able to characterize various tissue over a large bandwidth. They were able to characterize bones [47–49], thyroid tissues [50], adipose tissues [51], collagen [46,52], and elastin [53]. This groundwork was crucial in order to investigate the tissue composition of breast for example, which can help for diagnosis of cancerous tissue [54,55]. Finally, we can report that the latest reported system has also been used to monitor the thermal effect of Radio Frequency (RF) on tissues [56,57].

The previously reported systems were only composed of one channel, which can be a drawback when an image is required, like for performing mammography. Therefore, parallel to these developments, another system aimed at optical mammography was developed, based on a supercontinuum light generated in PCF and a 32-channel parallel detection [58]. This allowed to acquired image of the breast between 606 and 885 nm, and to extract hemoglobin, tissue saturation, lipid and water content, and scattering parameters of the tissue.

All the systems reported above were designed to collect spectral information about tissue, with a first application in breast cancer detection. Therefore, the acquisition time was not limited, and functional contrast was not explored. However, the potential of monitoring real time change in optical properties over a large bandwidth is quite appealing for various application, like brain monitoring [59]. Therefore, other systems were developed in order to achieve that goal. A system was developed at POLIMI based on a supercontinuum source generated in a PCF by a self-locking mode-locked Ti:Sapphire oscillator and a detection scheme based on an imaging spectrometer coupled to a 16-channel multianode PMT connected to a TCSPC board [60]. The fact that all the 16 wavelengths were captured at once enabled a fast acquisition and permitted to track dynamic variations in absorption and scattering spectra following hemodynamic changes [61]. The limitation of the detections scheme constraint the bandwidth of this system between 520 and 850 nm.

A similar approach was taken by a group based in Poland [62,63]. The system was based on a commercial SCL for the source, coupled to a 16-channel multianode PMT connected to a TCSPC board for the detection part. This system was used to follow a contrast agent (Indocyanine green (ICG)), which allows to estimate the cerebral blood perfusion. The same system can be used without ICG to monitor the intrinsic optical contrast [64]. Similarly, the author and colleagues used a TD-NIRS system based on a SCL filtered at 808 nm and on a detection scheme based on a single channel TCSPC to follow ICG bolus [65]. The novelty of this study was the fact that the TD-NIRS was coupled with a diffuse correlation spectroscopy system (DCS) [66]. The coupling of these two techniques allowed to retrieve absolute cerebral blood flow measurement in patients in the intensive care unit, showing that these systems could be used in a particularly difficult clinical environment. Moreover, the possibility to also measure blood perfusion is of great interest and might help in the adoption of the technique in the clinic.

Another potential detection scheme in order to collect parallel data is to use an Intensified CCD (ICCD) camera. Selb and collaborators used a commercial SCL combined with a ICCD camera to perform functional brain imaging with 2 wavelengths at a frequency of 3 Hz [67]. This system was an upgrade of a previously developed instrument based on pulsed Ti:Sapphire laser [68]. This source was tuneable but the switching time between wavelength was too slow to enable dual-wavelength functional imaging. Therefore, the authors report that the use of SCL unlocked this possibility with their detection scheme.

Similarly, Lange and collaborators described a TD-NIRS system developed to measure the human brain tissue physiology [69,70]. This system was based on commercial SCL for the emission and on an ICCD camera coupled with an imaging spectrometer in order to perform the spectral decomposition. This system allowed to retrieve the typical hemodynamic response, and preliminary results on the detection of oxCCO were also performed. The ability to retrieve oxCCO is exiting for brain applications, as it has been shown that this contrast can be more specific than the oxygenation, and that it can be an early biomarker of neonatal encephalopathy for example [7]. This possibility has been explored by the UCL team by developing a 4-channel 16 wavelengths TD-NIRS system in order to monitor both the oxygenation and oxCCO signal [24,71]. This system was based on time multiplexing, with a TCSPC detection scheme, but the fast-switching capabilities of the SCL coupled with AOTF allowed the acquisition of all the 16 wavelengths in less than 2 s. This system has also been used to evaluate the long-term reproducibility of the evaluation of cerebral tissue saturation in healthy adults with good reproducibility [72]. This system can be seen in Figure 2, and in an example of data in Figure 3.

Another approach that has been used using SCL sources is the development of non-contact systems. This can present several advantages to avoid issues attributed to sensor-tissue contact like skin compression and to obtain a reduction in measurement preparation time. A team at the Physikalisch-Technische Bundesanstalt (PTB) has developed a non-contact TD-NIRS system based on a commercial SCL and fast-gated SPAD to explore the human brain physiology [73–76]. At the time, the authors reported that the use of SCL permitted a shorter pulse width (<100 ps), an achievable output power considerably larger than picosecond diode lasers, and the possibility to quickly switch between two different wavelengths (i.e., on the µs to ms time scale). Moreover, the use of the SPAD in that system enables to reject the burst of early photons, which can improve the spatial resolution of the system at very short detector distances [77]. This process had been previously demonstrated by the POLIMI team that had develop a single channel TD-NIRS system based on SCL and a fast gated SPAD detector [78]. The POLIMI team has also worked on the modelling of the parameters of such detection schemes, in order to optimise their design [79].

The non-contact scheme is also very useful for pre-clinical applications. Indeed, several systems, based on SCL for the source, aiming at collecting physiological information of small animals, have been proposed. In the early 2000s, a system based on a home-made SC generation associated with an imaging spectrometer coupled with a streak camera was developed and used to monitor the cerebral hemodynamic of songbirds [80,81]. More recently, the UCL team have developed a system aiming at investigating both the cerebral hemodynamic and metabolic response (via oxCCO) of the exposed cortex of rodents [25]. In this work, a commercial SCL was used in combination with a dispersive prism, for the emission, and a sCMOS camera, as a detector, to record 11 images (11 wavelengths) of the exposed cortex in less than 0.3 s/wavelength. Here the recording was not time resolved, but the power of the laser and the ability to quickly switch between the wavelength had dictated the choice of this source. This system can be seen in Figure 2 and an example of data in Figure 3. Another approach can be to use spatial frequency domain imaging (SFDI), a wide-field, noncontact, model-based technique that can quantitatively assess absorption and scattering, on a pixel-by-pixel basis by calculating the modulation transfer function of structured light projected onto the tissue. This technique can be hyperspectral if a proper source is used. However, the system developed thus far was based on conventional broadband sources coupled with tunable filters, which limited their acquisition speed and spectral resolution. Torabzadeh and colleagues [82] applied this technique using the principles of the single-pixel compressive sensing. They used a commercial SCL coupled with a dispersive prism to achieve a final bandwidth 1000 spectral bands between 580 and 950 nm, which was larger than the previously developed systems. With this system, the authors were able to characterize the optical properties of a beef sample ex-vivo in 2D, and extract physiological information (i.e., hemoglobin content and fat and water content). The authors noted that the wavelength selection technique used was still slow (i.e., 150 s of acquisition time for a 4 cm × 6 cm), but that switching to an AOTF solution could greatly improve this speed. Using the same principle of the single-pixel compressive sensing, Farina and colleagues reported a TD-DOT instrument based on time-resolved single pixel camera [83]. Their approach was based on a SCL source filtered at 620 nm coupled with a digital micromirror device (DMD) to generate the spatial pattern. The time domain acquisition was based on TCSPC. Pian and colleagues used a similar approach but expended it to a broadband illumination and detection [84]. The authors reported that their system, aimed at fluorescence molecular tomography, benefitted for the commercial SCL source to perform hyperspectral excitation of the sample which offers a spectral information boost within the same data acquisition time compared to single wavelength excitation situations.

Another work aiming at improving the spatial resolution of TD-DOT was to investigate the effect of only considering early photons, which undergo fewer scattering events [85]. In this work, this approach has been tested using a commercial SCL together with a bandpass filter at 670 nm. It worth noting that the commercial version of this laser was modified by the manufacturer so that it had a shortened fibre compared to standard models, which reduced the pulse width to approximately 300 ps. This is important as the benefit of the gating of the early photons is highly dependent on the instrument response function (IRF) of the system. The authors reported that with this technique, and this instrument, a 64 to 84% image resolution could be achieved, which could be a great benefit for preclinical imaging with diffuse optics.

Novel algorithms can also be used in combination to TD-DOT instruments to recovers 3D images of the optical properties and physiological parameters. A team in Grenoble has explored the use of the Mellin-Laplace transform to reconstruct 3D images of the chromophores inside phantoms and for the non-invasive assessment of flap viability in rats' models. There instrumentation was based on commercial SCL, coupled with either an AOTF or an interferential filter, for the source and a TCPSC scheme for the detection [86,87].

TD-DOT has also been explored in humans, in order to reconstruct 2D or 3D maps of the optical properties and hemodynamic parameters. To this end, the UCL team had design MONSTIR II to perform tomographic brain imaging [28]. This system is based on a commercial SCL with an AOTF filtering and has 32 channels based on TCSPC. It was successfully used to scan healthy and ill infants in a clinical environment [88,89], an example of data produced by this system is provided in Figure 3. More recently, a new TD-DOT system based on a commercial SCL filtered by an AOTF, and a 32 × 32-pixel SPAD camera, has been developed by a team at the Biomedical Optics Research Laboratory at the University of Zurich [26,27,90]. This system operates at 2 wavelengths and at 11 sources points, which can be scanned in about 3 s. It is a big step forward compared to previously developed system, especially considering its size, as it is handheld. A picture of this instrument is reported in Figure 2.

Finally, all the instrument mentioned above were mostly based on the TD technique, or traditional white light illumination. We can note that we found one frequency domain (FD) system, that is based a commercial SCL to collect our system collects FD data at 170 wavelengths from 680 to 850 nm and allows to accurately measure absorption and scattering information about the tissue [91].

3.2. Methodology

We have seen that the SCL has been used to develop several systems, mainly aiming at characterising the optical properties of tissues over a large bandwidth or to non-invasively follow the oxygenation and/or metabolic changes both in humans and in preclinical models. Both of these capacities are extremely appealing for clinical applications. However, the transition to the clinical application of system based on SCL and more generally TD-NIRS/DOT is still happening at a slow pace. One of the reasons of the slow adoption of optical techniques is the lack of standards in the community. Indeed, standardisation is key in order to test all the systems on the same ground, and reenforce the trustworthiness of the technique. In the recent years, standardisation have been a main goal of the NIRS community, and several protocols have been developed in order to compare and test the capabilities of NIRS systems. The main produced protocols were the MEDPHOT [92], BIP [93], and nEUROpt [94]. It is out of the scope of this paper to describe these protocols in detail, but the cornerstones of all of these are to produce standard phantoms, well characterized spectrally in terms of absorption and scattering coefficients, in order to be able to quantitatively compare different systems or methods. In this matter, SCL based systems were extensively used to characterize the material used to produce these phantoms and the actual final phantoms used as standard. These optical phantoms can either be solid (easier to store and stable over a long period of time) or liquid (easier to precisely tune the optical properties of the solution and to adjust it dynamically). For the liquid phantoms, the core principle is to use a fatty solution to control the scattering coefficient of the solution, and ink to control their absorption properties. Several recipes have been tested, like using Agar and Triton [95], but the most common recipe to date is to use a combination of water, intralipid and Indian ink. This choice has arisen after a careful characterization of both intralipid and Indian ink, principally with instrument based on SCL [96–100]. We can note that for the precise optical characterisation of liquid, techniques based on integrating sphere are often used. However, this methodology cannot be applied for large solid phantoms. In this matter, TD-NIRS has proved a good methodology to accurately estimates the optical properties. For example, in 2010, Bouchard and colleagues used a TD-NIRS setup based on a SCL source filtered at 610 nm in order to estimate the optical properties of phantom with an absolute error estimates of 0.01 cm^{-1} (11.3%) and 0.67 cm^{-1} (6.8%) for the absorption coefficient and reduced scattering coefficient, respectively [101].

On top of designing phantom able to mimic the background optical properties of tissues, some methods have emerged to mimic a perturbation of the absorption coefficient within a homogeneous medium. To that end, one can either use a liquid phantom for the homogeneous medium, and a small black PVC target for the perturbation. A protocol has been designed and it is possible to precisely set the absorption perturbation value based on the size of the black PVC inclusion [94]. This protocol has been validated with Monte Carlo simulations and in-situ using a system based on SCL [102]. A similar phantom based on a completely solid phantom, with a movable solid rod, has also been designed and characterised [103]. Lastly, some phantoms have also been characterized in order to be a tool to evaluate quantitatively the responsivity of NIRS systems [104].

Finally, we can also mention new approaches based on digital phantoms. Basically, rather than physically simulating the process of light propagation in tissue, the digital phantom provides the detector with light signals mimicking the signals obtained in-vivo. Such systems based on an integrating sphere and several light sources, including a commercial SCL, have been proposed to spectrally characterise and calibration optical systems [105]. More recently, a digital phantom has been developed to mimic TD-NIRS signal acquisition, and the authors used various sources and detectors in order to test this approach, including a SCL [106]. One other important component to optically characterize is the optode holders used to secure the optical fibres to the patient. In a recent study, Amendola and colleagues used a system previously developed to evaluate the optical properties of fruit [107] (based on a commercial SCL and a filter wheel to select 14 spectral band in the range 550 to 940 nm) to spectrally characterised poly lactic acid (PLA), a material used for

3D printing [108]. As 3D printing is more and more common in order to produce probe holders, it is important to optically characterise the material used in order to avoid any unwanted effects on the measurement provoked by light interaction with the material. In that study, the authors concluded that the different material tested were not optically the same, and that characterisation was important before their use.

The development of all these phantoms has provided a good framework for the developers to compare their systems and methods in order to provide robust clinical information. Regarding the instrumentation, a lot of effort are currently being made in order to improve the detection scheme of TD-NIRS. To that end, SCL have been a source of choice to test new detectors like the promising fast silicon photomultiplier (SiPM) which drastically improve light harvesting compared to the old PMTs [109–111]. SCL based systems have also been used to characterise novel bio-compatible fibres that can be implanted in the patient with potential use in the monitoring of the evolution of the physiology after a surgical intervention or in photodynamic therapy (PDT) [112,113].

Regarding the methodology, several new data processing techniques have been explored and tested in conjunction with SCL. Indeed, system based on SCL can collect multidimensional data that can be coupled together in order to improve the accuracy of the data, reduce the noise or explore new contrast. One of the first work regarding this matter dates from 2006, where D'Andrea and colleagues, showed that one could increase the robustness of the determination of the chromophore's concentrations in tissues (hemoglobin, water, lipid) by using a spectral constraint during the fitting procedure [114]. This showed the strength of using the spectral dimension coupled with the DTOF, which is accessible when using SCL. This method has also been used to monitor absorption changes in a layered diffusive medium [115], which is relevant in the monitoring of brain activation for example. Similar approaches were explored in the same group in order to accurately monitor the spectral changes in absorption coefficients of turbid media [116].

One can also use the spatial dimension in order to enhance the amount of information recorded, by recording data from multiple source-detector distances. This approach has been recently tested and it has been shown that coupling the spatial dimension with the DTOF could increase the accuracy of the estimation of the optical properties [117–119]. Another interesting use of the spatial dimension is the self-calibrating method for TD-NIRS, which uses the spatial dimension in order to avoid the measurement of the IRF, that is needed to remove the effect of the instrument from the response of the tissue [120]. The characterisation of the IRF necessitates an extra step that can be a burden in a clinical environment. Therefore, this method could facilitate the use of TD-NIRS in the clinic. Finally, we can also report that an approach combining the spatial and spectral dimension proved to also improve the accuracy of the results of CW-NIRS. This has been tested recently, especially with blood phantoms and compared to the results of a TD-NIRS instrument based on a SCL source [121].

The large amount of data collected by TD-NIRS also enables different data processing scheme to extract the relevant information. Therefore, there is a need to properly compare all the available methods in order to evaluate their strength and weaknesses. This work has recently been undertaken in order to compare the moment and time windowing techniques [122,123]. Having a deep understanding of all the data processing method is also crucial so the proper technique can be used depending on the application.

Several multi-centre initiatives have recently promoted this standardisation effort to compare instruments and algorithms. To that end, partners from the BitMap network (http://www.bitmap-itn.eu/, accessed date: 1 February 2021) have started comparing instruments from different institutions all over Europe, by using the same sets of solid phantoms from the 3 main protocols [124,125]. Moreover, several centres in Europe have used their instruments (several based on SCL) on 9 subjects, to study the inter-subject variability of the optical properties of the human head measured by several instruments [126]. They could show that the inter-subject variability was significant, with a big effect of the technique used (either CW or TD) because of their different depth sensitivity, which in turn affects the averaged optical properties retrieved. Therefore, it is evident that all the efforts to precisely characterized instruments and methods will have a huge impact on the precision of the optical measurement of tissue parameters.

Finally, the use of SCL can help to explore new avenues in diffuse optics. The main one is to go above the "therapeutical window" in the second (1100 nm to 1350 nm) and the third (1600 to 1870 nm) near-infrared optical window. On top of the previously reported works that expand the bandwidth of TD-NIRS systems up to 1700 nm, Sordillo and colleagues reported the use of a commercial SCL source, filtered with a bandpass and long pass filters to target the second and third NIR windows, coupled with an IR-CCD camera, to acquire transmission images of 3 targets embedded in chicken tissue of various thickness [127]. They were able to distinguish the targets up to a depth of 10 mm, which was not possible when using the same setup but with a traditional lamp source. These results are promising in order to implement transmission measurement, especially for preclinical imaging.

As we have seen previously, the use of these long NIR wavelength is useful to resolve more chromophores like collagen. It is also promising to resolve glucose, which could be a true benefit for several clinical applications like monitoring diabetes [128], or monitoring brain injuries [129] or neonatal encephalopathy [130]. Once again, in this wavelength range, the power delivered by SCL has proved efficient to monitor the glucose contrast in the NIR [131,132].

Finally, a tentative to non-invasively probe the lungs with a TD-NIRS system based on SCL source was reported [133]. The measurements were performed on three subjects, and spectra from 600 to 1100 nm could be acquired. Here, the depth sensitivity of a TD-NIRS is essential and this application shows that instruments based on that technology could be used to non-invasively probes tissues previously thought out of reach.

Table 2. Table of the literature review of the use of SC lasers in biomedical diffuse optics. The system used in each study are described more in detail in Table 1 and referred to as "system ID". μ_a: absorption coefficient, μ'_s: reduced scattering coefficient.

Publication	Year	System ID	Category of Study	Target of Study	Reported Quantities
S. Andersson-Engels et al. [29]	1993	1	System development	Multispectral tissue characterisation	μ_a
af Klinteberg et al. [30]	1995	1	Optical properties estimation	Breast tissue examination	μ_a, μ'_s
Bassi et al. [60]	2004	2	System development	Phantoms and in vivo validation measurements	μ_a, μ'_s
Abrahamsson et al. [32]	2004	3	System development	Sample characterisation	μ_a, μ'_s
Swartling et al. [61]	2005	3	System development	Phantoms and in vivo validation measurements	μ_a, μ'_s, [HbT], StO_2
Ramstein et al. [81]	2005	4	System development	Optical properties in vivo monitoring of songbird brain	μ_a, μ'_s
D'Andrea et al. [114]	2006	2	Methodology	Validation of spectral fitting analysis	μ_a, μ'_s, H_2O, Water Content Lipid Content, [HbO$_2$], [HHb], [HbT], StO_2
Bassi et al. [58]	2006	2	System development	Optical mammography	μ_a, μ'_s, H_2O, Lipid Content, [HbT], StO_2
Bassi et al. [38]	2007	6	System development	Phantoms and in vivo breast validation	μ_a, μ'_s, H_2O, Lipid Content, [HbO$_2$], [HHb], [HbT], StO_2
Vignal et al. [134]	2008	4	Application	In vivo measurement of brain hemodynamic changes in songbird	[HbO$_2$], [HHb], [HbT]
Farina et al. [40]	2009	6	Methodology	Study and correction of bandpass effects in TD spectroscopy	μ_a
Taroni et al. [39]	2009	6	System development	In vivo measurements of breast tissue	μ_a, μ'_s, Water Content, Lipid Content, Collagen Content, [HbT], StO_2
Svensson et al. [42]	2009	7	System development	Validation on phantoms	μ_a, μ'_s
Valim et al. [85]	2010	8	Methodology	Study of PDSF in phantoms	Photon density sensitivity function (PDSF)
Bouchard et al. [101]	2010	9	Methodology	Characterisation of tissue-mimicking phantoms	n, g, μ_a, μ'_s
Pifferi et al. [116]	2010	15	Methodology	Data processing	$\Delta\mu_a$
Taroni et al. [52]	2010	15	Optical properties estimation	Characterisation of collagen optical properties	μ_a, μ'_s
Giusto et al. [115]	2010	2	Methodology	Data Processing	μ_a, μ'_s, [HbO$_2$], [HHb]
Dalla Mora et al. [78]	2010	6	Methodology	Electronic development	μ_a, μ'_s
Mottin et al. [80]	2011	4	Application	In vivo study of brain oxygen uncoupling/recoupling in songbirds	[HbO$_2$], [HHb]
Mazurenka et al. [73]	2011	10	System development	Non-contact TD-NIRS	Contrast
Arnesano et al. [91]	2012	11	System development	FD spectroscopy for tissue imaging	μ_a, μ'_s
Spinelli et al. [97]	2012	Multiple systems	Optical properties estimation	Characterisation of liquid phantoms	Intrinsic absorption coefficient, Intrinsic reduced scattering coefficient
Bargigia et al. [44]	2012	13	System development	Characterisation on lipids	μ_a, μ'_s
Gerega et al. [63]	2012	12	Methodology	TD-NIRS with ICG	Fluorescence of ICG
Bargigia et al. [43]	2012	15	System development	Bandwidth up to 1700 nm	μ_a, μ'_s

Table 2. Cont.

Publication	Year	System ID	Category of Study	Target of Study	Reported Quantities
Xu et al. [105]	2012	Laser not specified	Methodology	Digital phantom characterisation	StO_2
Wang et al. [96]	2012	16	System development	Liquid optical phantom characterisation in the second and third optical window	g, μ_a, μ'_s
Selb et al. [67]	2013	14	System development	Functional brain imaging	$\Delta[HbO_2], \Delta[HHb]$
Bargigia et al. [45]	2013	13	System development	In vivo measurements of forearm and breast	Water Content, Lipid Content, Collagen Content
Farina et al. [41]	2013	6	Methodology	Comparison of approaches for spectral selection	μ_a, μ'_s
Mazurenka et al. [75]	2013	26	System development	Non-contact system	$\Delta[HbO_2], \Delta[HHb]$
Wabnitz et al. [135]	2013	Multiple instruments	Methodology	multi-laboratory study to assess the performance of time-domain optical brain imagers	μ_a, μ'_s
Quarto et al. [95]	2013	15	Methodology	Phantom characterisation	μ_a, μ'_s
Aernouts et al. [98]	2013	16	Optical properties estimation	Phantom characterisation	g, μ_a, μ'_s
Quarto et al. [133]	2013	15	Methodology	In vivo optical diagnostics of lung conditions and diseases	μ_a, μ'_s
Aernouts et al. [99]	2014	16	Optical properties estimation	Phantom characterisation	g, μ_a, μ'_s
Spinelli et al. [100]	2014	6	Optical properties estimation	Phantom characterisation	μ_a, μ'_s
Cooper et al. [28]	2014	17	System development	Brain TD-DOT	μ_a, μ'_s
Farina et al. [126]	2014	Multiple instruments	Optical properties estimation	Brain Tissue-characterisation	μ_a, μ'_s
Wabnitz et al. [93]	2014	17	Methodology	Instrumental performance protocol	Instrument parameters
Wabnitz et al. [94]	2014	17	Methodology	Instrumental performance protocol	Instrument parameters, μ_a
Martelli et al. [102]	2014	18	Methodology	Phantom characterisation	μ_a, μ'_s
Taroni et al. [55]	2015	6	Optical properties estimation	In vivo quantification of collagen in breast tissue	Water Content, Lipid Content, Collagen Content, Collagen index, [HbT], StO_2
Lange et al. [70]	2015	19	System development	Functional brain monitoring	$\Delta[HbO_2], \Delta[HHb], \Delta[oxCCO]$
Farina et al. [83]	2015	20	System development	TD-DOT/FMT	Fluorescence
Contini et al. [79]	2015	21	Methodology	Time-gated measurements on tissue phantoms	Contrast
Della Mora et al. [109]	2015	22	Methodology	Testing of a SiPM	μ_a, μ'_s
Pifferi et al. [103]	2015	15	Methodology	Phantom characterisation	μ_a, μ'_s
Martinenghi et al. [110]	2015	15	Methodology	Characterisation of SiPM detectors	Instrument parameters
Dempsey et al. [88]	2015	17	Methodology	Whole-head TD-DOT in neonates	μ_a, μ'_s
Sordillo et al. [127]	2015	23	Methodology	Deep-tissue, optical properties monitoring	μ_a

Table 2. *Cont.*

Publication	Year	System ID	Category of Study	Target of Study	Reported Quantities
Konugolu Venkata Sekar et al. [47]	2015	24	Optical properties estimation	In vivo measurement of optical properties of bone	μ_a, μ'_s, Water Content, Lipid Content, Collagen Content, [HbO$_2$], [HHb], [HbT], StO$_2$
Konugolu Venkata Sekar et al. [23]	2016	24	Optical properties estimation	In vivo human tissues measurements	μ_a, μ'_s, H$_2$O, Lipid, Collagen, [HbO$_2$], [HHb], [HbT], StO$_2$
Di Sieno et al. [76]	2016	25	System development	Validation on phantoms	Instrument parameters
Wabnitz et al. [104]	2016	26	Optical properties estimation	Phantoms characterisation	μ_a, μ'_s
Konugolu Venkata Sekar et al. [49]	2016	24	Optical properties estimation	In vivo measurement of optical properties of bone	μ_a, μ'_s, Water Content, Lipid Content, Collagen Content, [HbO$_2$], [HHb], StO$_2$
Konugolu Venkata Sekar et al. [48]	2016	24	Optical properties estimation	In vivo measurement of optical properties of bone	μ_a, μ'_s, Water Content, Lipid Content, Collagen Content, [HbO$_2$], [HHb], [HbT], StO$_2$
Martinenghi et al. [111]	2016	13	Methodology	Characterisation of SiPM detectors	Instrument parameters
Di Sieno et al. [87]	2016	27	System development	In vivo assessment of flap viability	[HbO$_2$], [HHb]
Zouaoui et al. [86]	2017	22	Methodology	Validation of chromophore decomposition algorithm	Dyes content
Konugolu Venkata Sekar et al. [46]	2017	24	Optical properties estimation	In vivo measurement of optical properties of collagen	μ_a Collagen
Wabnitz et al. [74]	2017	27	Methodology	Non-contact TD brain imaging	Intensity Contrast
Di Sieno et al. [112]	2017	24	Methodology	Characterisation of bioresorbable fibres	μ_a, μ'_s
Konugolu Venkata Sekar et al. [53]	2017	24	Optical properties estimation	In vivo measurement of optical properties of elastin	μ_a and μ'_s Elastin
Jiang et al. [90]	2017	39	Methodology	Data Processing—GPU	μ_a, μ'_s
Konugolu Venkata Sekar et al. [50]	2018	24	Optical properties estimation	In vivo chromophore characterisation of thyroid	μ_a, μ'_s
Lange et al. [69]	2018	19	System development	In vivo monitoring of brain physiological changes in humans	Δ[HbO$_2$], Δ[HHb]
Pian et al. [84]	2018	29	System development	Validation on phantoms	μ_a
Gerega et al. [62]	2018	30	Application	assessment of intracerebral and extracerebral absorption changes	Δ[ICG]
He et al. [65]	2018	31	Application	continuous monitoring of absolute cerebral blood flow (CBF) in adult human patients	CBF
Della Mora et al. [113]	2018	15	Methodology	bioresorbable optical fibers	Contrast, μ_a, μ'_s
Laura Dempsey [89]	2018	17	System development	Brain TD-DOT	[HbO$_2$], [HHb]
Liu et al. [131]	2018	28	Methodology	Glucose monitoring	[Glucose]
Wabnitz et al. [106]	2019	32	Methodology	Validation of digital phantom	Phantom parameters and basic responses of the instrument to it

Table 2. Cont.

Publication	Year	System ID	Category of Study	Target of Study	Reported Quantities
Fuglerud et al. [132]	2019	33	Methodology	Glucose sensing in blood	[Glucose]
Torabzadeh et al. [82]	2019	34	System development	Spatial FD HIS on ex vivo beef sample	μ_a, μ'_s, Water Content, lipid Content, [HbO$_2$], [HHb], [MHb]
Lange et al. [24]	2019	35	System development	Validation on phantoms	μ_a, μ'_s, [HbO$_2$], [HHb], [oxCCO]
Ferocino et al. [54]	2019	24	Methodology	Validation on phantoms of TD-NIRs reconstruction algorithm	μ_a, μ'_s
Lange et al. [72]	2019	35	Application	Reproducibility analysis of cerebral oxygenation measured with TD-NIRS	[HbO$_2$], [HHb], StO$_2$
Yang et al. [118]	2019	36	Methodology	Validation on phantoms of a multivariate TD-SD algorithm	μ_a, μ'_s
Yang et al. [117]	2019	36	Methodology	Validation on phantoms of a multivariate TD-SD algorithm	μ_a, μ'_s
Ferocino et al. [136]	2019	24	Methodology	Validation on meat samples of TD-NIRs reconstruction algorithm	[HbO$_2$]
Wojtkiewicz et al. [120]	2019	30	Methodology	Validation on phantoms and in vivo of a self-calibrating TD algorithm	μ_a, μ'_s, [HbO$_2$], [HHb]
Sudakou et al. [64]	2019	30	System development	Multi wavelength TD-NIRS system for brain monitoring	[HbO$_2$], [HHb], [HbT]
Wabnitz et al. [122]	2020	17	Methodology	Depth-selective analysis in TD optical brain imaging	μ_a, μ'_s
Lanka et al. [51]	2020	24	Optical properties estimation	In vivo measurement of optical properties of adipose tissue	μ_a, μ'_s, Water Content, Lipid Content, Collagen Content, [HbO$_2$], [HHb], [HbT], StO$_2$
Sudakou et al. [123]	2020	37	Methodology	Performance of measurands in TD optical brain imaging	μ_a, μ'_s
Yang et al. [119]	2020	32	Methodology	Space-enhanced TD diffuse optics in two-layered structures	μ_a, μ'_s
Lanka et al. [56]	2020	24	Methodology	Monitoring of thermal treatment in biological tissues	μ_a, μ'_s
Amendola et al. [108]	2020	24	Methodology	Effect of the 3d printed material on raw data	Photon Counts
Jiang et al. [26]	2020	39	System development	Novel TD-NIRS system based on SPAD camera	μ_a, μ'_s
Jiang et al. [27]	2020	39	Methodology	Image reconstruction for TD-NIRS system based on SPAD system	μ_a
Kovacsova et al. [121]	2021	35	Methodology	Validation of broadband oximetry algorithm	μ_a, μ'_s, StO$_2$
Giannoni et al. [25]	2021	38	System development	HSI of in vivo hemoglobin and CCO in the exposed cortex of mice	Δ[HbO$_2$], Δ[HHb], Δ[oxCCO]

4. Discussion

We have summarized the use of SCL sources in biomedical diffuse optics. Historically, these sources were allowed to develop TD-NIRS system as they could deliver a pulsed coherent light at several MHz with narrow pulse width in order to reduce the IRF [137], and high power, of several mW/Wavelength, which were characteristically difficult to achieve in the early 1990s. Moreover, the development of commercially available compact SCL in the 2000s also helped the development of the use of these sources, and we have reported that more companies (see Figure 1) are now able to provide such sources.

The main advantage of these sources is that they make it easier to explore more wavelength, enabling a multispectral or even broadband or hyperspectral measurement. Several measurement strategies can be implemented in order to do so. The first one is to use the white light as a source and achieve the spectral unmixing at the detection stage. The first available option to do so was to use an imaging spectrometer coupled with a streak camera, which achieve very high temporal resolution (in terms of arrival time of photons). However, this solution was bulky, and the sensitivity of these camera was low compared to the newest detection technologies. The same method can be used by either coupling the spectrometer with an ICCD camera, or a 16-channel TCSPC. This approach of performing the spectral unmixing on the detection can achieve faster measurement since no spectral switching mechanism is employed. However, the resolution of these approaches, either spectrally or temporally, can be limited. For example, typical ICCD cameras have a gate width of 200 ps, which limits the temporal resolution of the DTOF. On the other end, the 16-channel TCSPC system used by Sudakou and colleagues [64] allows spectral bands of 12.5 nm, limiting the spectral resolution. The other option to perform the spectral unmixing is to do a sequential acquisition, by filtering the white light on the source side. To do so, two main approach are used, (1) using an AOTF, with the ability of fast switching (few microseconds) but with a potential degradation of the spectral response (i.e., side lobs), and (2) using a dispersing prism which can be mounted on a rotating axis, which can achieve better spectral performances but at the cost of a slower switching time. Therefore, the choice of the instrumentation depends on the end application, and trade-off needs to be made between spectral quality and acquisition speed. Whatever the requirement, we have seen that SCL can be used and coupled with various type of instrumentation in order to accommodate to the requirements of the applications.

From an application point of view, the ability to monitor a large number of several wavelengths has several advantages. First of all, it enables to provides a true spectroscopic analysis, both in terms of absorption and scattering. This is extremely appealing for cancer application, where this type of "optical biopsy", enables to distinguish between healthy and cancerous tissue. This type of application has been extensively used in breast cancer [138,139], and more recently, thyroid applications [50,140]. In this type of application, where the spectral quality is the most important criteria, the second instrumental approach, based on spectral unmixing with a dispersing prism, was used. Secondly, the first instrumental approach, based on spectral unmixing at the detection stage, or the second instrumental approach using ATOF, give the possibility to acquire several wavelengths, either parallelly, or with a fast switching, in a time scale compatible with functional imaging. With these approaches, several authors have explicitly noted that the adoption of SCL enabled them to design or update existing systems, in order to retrieve dynamic physiological information [67,75].

The large number of wavelengths enabled by SCL also give the possibility to go beyond the traditional contrasts, like the hemodynamic one, in order to get information about metabolism for example, by extracting information about more chromophores, like oxCCO [7,24]. We can also note that beyond the intrinsic optical signal, a contrast agent, like ICG, can also be used in order to get information on tissue perfusion. This has notably been extensively used to monitor cerebral perfusion, and the SCL has also proved to be a suitable light source for these applications, even used in extremely complicated clinical settings like ICUs [65].

From a historical point of view, we can note that the development of commercial fibre also largely helped with the adoption of that technology. Indeed, out of the 35 different systems used in the reviewed paper, only 4 (less than 12%) are home-made. They correspond to the system developed before 2010. Past that date, all systems reviewed used a commercial source. We can also see the increase number of papers since the adoption of the commercial sources, with a number of papers published per year roughly doubling from that date. One of the main advantages reported by the authors when they adopted commercial SCL was their relative compactness, compared to the initial development of SC generation. This can be seen in Figure 2, with systems able to be mounted on trolley compatible with the clinical environment. However, the use of these lasers in actual clinical studies remains marginal. In our recent review [141], which has explored the use of TD-NIRS for clinical applications, less than 4% of the 52 papers reviewed were using a system based on a SCL source. Indeed, despite their advantages, a few drawbacks still hindered the adoption of SCL as a standard source. The first one is the cost which, despite a significant decrease in the recent years, remains high (i.e., more than 20,000 pounds for a SCL with several watts of power, enabling a final power of at least 1 mW per wavelength). The second main disadvantage is the warmup time, and the overall stability of these sources. Indeed, the stability of the output can be a concern, but the use of a reference arm can solve this issue [23]. This of course comes at the cost of a more complicated and bulkier instrument. Regarding the warmup time, typically, 1 h is required so the instrument reach thermal equilibrium, which can be too long for certain clinical applications. Some recent TD-NIRS systems based on pulsed laser diode have reported a warmup time of only 15 min, which is way more advantageous in a clinical setting [142]. Finally, even though the novel commercial SCL are more compact than in the early days, their size is still significantly bigger than traditional pulsed laser diode, which limit the reduction of the overall instrument size. Therefore, this can also slow down the adoption of these systems, as space are often very limited in busy clinical environment like ICUs.

These drawbacks are less of an issue for the preclinical settings as the environment is way less constrained. Therefore, the great potential of applications based on SCL outweighs its current main drawbacks, and several instruments based on SCL have been developed for preclinical imaging. The interested reader can refer to the recent review by Bérubé-Lauzière and colleagues, which explore more particularly the use of DOT in preclinical settings [143]. It worth noting that these systems are non-contact, and that this particular detection approach has also been explored for human imaging. Here, having an extremely narrow pulse, like the one provided by SCL, is of great interest as one can take advantage of the null-source approach [77]. Even if these approaches are less common, they can have potential great applications for perioperative measurements, or when the patient is difficult to access, and represent a promising avenue.

The above-mentioned drawbacks are also less problematic in a typical lab setting. SCL are a great tool for teams aiming at instrumental and methodological developments. In the reviewed papers, 33% were aimed at the initial system developments, and 18% and 44% were focused on optical tissue estimations or methodological developments, respectively. Only 5% of the reported studies were focused on pure applications, like tissue oxygenation estimation or cancer monitoring. Indeed, the availability of these SCL sources in teams focused on methodological and instrumental developments have pushed their used to test new possibilities and enhance the reliability of the system by promoting standardization. It is worth mentioning that having a SCL is not mandatory in a lot of settings, and that these sources were used as they were available in most of the groups working on instrumental and methodological developments. Indeed, in the case of a CW system, we have seen that SCL systems were used to provide a high number of wavelengths. In that case, other broadband sources are available, like Tungsten Halogen Light Sources (THLS) or like the Laser-Driven Light Sources (LDLS). The main disadvantage of the THLS is the low power density/wavelength, compared to coherent sources, which can limit their possibilities in biomedical diffuse optics. However, we can still report that THLS were successfully used to developed simple CW instruments [144,145]. On the contrary, the novel LDLS are of interest as they can produce a stable, high power broadband light. This technology is still relatively new and, to our knowledge, has not been used in biomedical diffuse optics yet. However, its attractive characteristics could be of interest for developing CW biomedical diffuse optics systems. The interested reader can refer to review [146] for more details. Finally, we can note that designing a multi-wavelengths CW system by adding up several single wavelengths light sources, like LEDs, is possible, but it is limited to a low number of wavelengths as the bulkiness and cost of the systems would rapidly increase with the number of wavelengths. In the case of TD systems, the choice of the light source is also largely dictated by the number of wavelengths needed, as can be seen in Table 3, that summarizes the relative advantages and disadvantages of single wavelength laser diode sources versus SCL in two cases: (1) low and (2) high number of wavelengths for TD systems. The use of single wavelength laser diode sources is indeed well adapted when a low number of wavelengths is required, as these sources are compact and relatively not expensive regarding the SCL ones. However, if one wants to design a truly spectroscopic system, with a high number of wavelengths required, these advantages became less evident as, similarly to the CW case, the bulkiness and cost of the system increase as function as the number of wavelengths. This is even more pronounced for the TD cases as the electronics are more complex. Finally, we can mention that if one wants to focus on methodological development, when specific wavelengths are still not defined, the flexibility of SCL is then evident as this choice does not have to be made from the start of the designing process, and not all the wavelengths are available commercially with laser diodes. Therefore, even though other light sources with characteristics compatible with diffuse optics are available, the high power, broadband spectrum, and fast switching capabilities of SCL makes them a source of choice, sufficiently versatile to be able to explore various avenues without source limitations.

Table 3. Main relative advantages and drawbacks of single wavelength laser diode sources and SCL as function as the number of wavelengths used for TD systems. (+ advantages / − disadvantages). FW: Few Wavelength, HNW: High number of Wavelengths.

	Single Wavelength Sources		Supercontinuum Laser	
	Few Wavelengths	High number of Wavelengths	Few Wavelengths	High Number of Wavelengths
Cost	++	−−	−−	+
Stability	+	+	−	−
Compactness	++	−−	−−	+
Wavelength Choice	Limited	Limited	Unlimited	Unlimited
Overall	+++	−−	−−	++

This spectral flexibility offered by SCL has indeed been a true advantage regarding the standardization efforts, giving the ability to optically characterize over a large bandwidth material and tissue. Phantom materials, like Intralipid or Indian ink, have been able to be precisely characterized using SCL, enabling to produce reproducible recipes for liquid phantoms, or to produces reliable solid phantoms. This now gives the possibility to accurately and quantitatively test and compare newly developed instruments and algorithms. We can note the effort undertaken by the BitMap project that have started comparing instruments, from different institutions all over Europe, using the same sets of solid phantoms [124,125].

SCL can also be used as companions to develop new electronic components. Indeed, one of the big instrumental development in the recent year have been the refinement of the detection scheme. Especially, a lot of improvement have been seen in novel solid state detectors [147] which enable to boost light harvesting detectors electronics. The development of gated detector [148] also enables techniques like null source distance to be practically implemented, which can improve the resolution and sensitivity of the technique [77]. In these works, the availability of SCL sources enabled to perform a precise characterisation of these detectors in situ, both in terms of temporal resolution, thanks to the short pulse width of the SCL, and in terms of spectral responsivity over a large bandwidth. The combination of the SCL capabilities with these new detectors can notably boost the capabilities of TD-NIR instrument, overcoming some current limitations like, for example, the penetration depth [22,149].

The inherent ability of SCL sources to construct systems gathering multidimensional information, i.e., spatial/spectral/temporal, also makes them a perfect tool to test novel algorithms able to exploit this large amount of data. The recent works by Yang and colleagues [117–119] show the advantages of using multi-dimensional datasets, by enhancing the accuracy of the optical properties estimation of tissues by using simultaneously the temporal and spatial dimensions. Kovacsova and colleagues [121] also showed this utility, here combining the spectral and the spatial dimensions. It worth noting that this work is based on broadband CW-NIRS, but that the results of this algorithm has been tested against a TD-NIRS instrument based on SCL as a source. Combining all the dimensions available is certainly a really exiting avenue for the field of diffuse optics, to make the system even more robust and precise.

Finally, we can mention that in the recent years, progress has also been made in individual pulsed laser source, which now achieve several 10th of mW and a pulse width shorter than 100 ps. A good example of the uses of these sources can be found in [150], where an 8 wavelengths TD-NIRS system, compatible for breast imaging for example, has been developed. This paves the way on the use of these sources to enable miniaturisation of TD-NIRS instruments, making them truly compatible with the clinic. These sources could then replace the SCL in clinical settings. However, depending on the application and the chromophores targeted, the wavelength selection is a process that requires some investigations in order to balance the system complexity, and the possible crosstalk effects between the chosen wavelengths. Therefore, systems based on SCL able to easily explore various combinations of wavelengths are once more extremely useful. Lastly, the flexibility of these systems also allows to explore new horizons and applications area, like we have seen with exploring contrast above the classical therapeutic windows (i.e., above 1000 nm) [46], or to explore new organs, like lungs [133]. Therefore, even though the main drawbacks of SCL in terms of absolute cost, size, and stability might prevent their use on a wide scale in the clinical world, their main advantages in terms of power, wavelength choice, and relatively low cost for high number of wavelengths is likely to still push their use in the labs to drive forward the clinical innovation in biomedical diffuse optics.

5. Conclusions

We have seen that the use of SCL drove the developments in biomedical diffuse optics, and particularly in TD-NIRS. First of all, it is a tool of choice to estimate the optical properties of tissues and phantom material over a large bandwidth. This knowledge is crucial in order to develop a standardized method, and to provide a-priori information used in the calculation of in vivo chromophores concentration for example. Moreover, the high spectral power combined with the ability to easily and quickly select wavelength make SCL suitable not only for in vivo tissue characterization, and application like breast cancer monitoring, but also to follow fast dynamic physiological processes like cerebral hemodynamic. The large number of wavelength available in the systems based on SCL (several systems reported parallel or quasi-parallel acquisition of up to 16 wavelengths) not only enables to refine the precision of the measurement, but also provides extra information about different processes like metabolism. These sources are also relevant to design instrument aiming at non-contact scanning, which make them also a good candidate for preclinical applications. In conclusion, SCL are a valuable tool at every step of the developmental and translational work, from fundamental characterization to preclinical and clinical use, and we have no doubt that it will still be an important brick to keep driving the innovation in biomedical diffuse optics.

Author Contributions: F.L., L.G. and I.T. conceived and designed the study. F.L. conducted the literature search and drafted the first version of the paper. L.G. created Tables 1 and 2. All authors have read and agreed to the published version of the manuscript.

Funding: This research was funded by the Medical Research Council (MR/S003134/1).

Institutional Review Board Statement: Not applicable.

Informed Consent Statement: Not applicable.

Conflicts of Interest: The authors declare no conflict of interest. The funders had no role in the design of the study; in the collection, analyses, or interpretation of data; in the writing of the manuscript, or in the decision to publish the results.

References

1. Elwell, C.E.; Cooper, C.E. Making light work: Illuminating the future of biomedical optics. *Philos. Trans. R. Soc. A Math. Phys. Eng. Sci.* **2011**, *369*, 4358–4379. [CrossRef] [PubMed]
2. Maniewsk, R.; Liebert, A.; Kacprzak, M.; Zbieć, A. Selected applications of near infrared optical methods in medical diagnosis. *OptoElectron. Rev.* **2004**, *12*, 255–262.
3. Martelli, F.; Binzoni, T.; Pifferi, A.; Spinelli, L.; Farina, A.; Torricelli, A. There's plenty of light at the bottom: Statistics of photon penetration depth in random media. *Sci. Rep.* **2016**, *6*, 27057. [CrossRef] [PubMed]
4. Wolf, M.; Ferrari, M.; Quaresima, V. Progress of near-infrared spectroscopy and topography for brain and muscle clinical applications. *J. Biomed. Opt.* **2007**, *12*, 62104.
5. Scholkmann, F.; Kleiser, S.; Metz, A.J.; Zimmermann, R.; Mata Pavia, J.; Wolf, U.; Wolf, M. A review on continuous wave functional near-infrared spectroscopy and imaging instrumentation and methodology. *Neuroimage* **2014**, *85*, 6–27. [CrossRef] [PubMed]
6. Yeganeh, H.Z.; Toronov, V.; Elliott, J.T.; Diop, M.; Lee, T.-Y.; St Lawrence, K. Broadband continuous-wave technique to measure baseline values and changes in the tissue chromophore concentrations. *Biomed. Opt. Express* **2012**, *3*, 2761–2770. [CrossRef] [PubMed]
7. Bale, G.; Elwell, C.E.; Tachtsidis, I. From Jöbsis to the present day: A review of clinical near-infrared spectroscopy measurements of cerebral cytochrome-c-oxidase. *J. Biomed. Opt.* **2016**, *21*, 091307. [CrossRef]
8. Yamada, Y.; Suzuki, H.; Yamashita, Y. Time-Domain Near-Infrared Spectroscopy and Imaging: A Review. *Appl. Sci.* **2019**, *9*, 1127. [CrossRef]
9. Grosenick, D.; Wabnitz, H.; Macdonald, R. Diffuse near-infrared imaging of tissue with picosecond time resolution. *Biomed. Eng. Biomed. Tech.* **2018**, *63*, 511–518. [CrossRef] [PubMed]
10. Torricelli, A.; Contini, D.; Pifferi, A.; Caffini, M.; Re, R.; Zucchelli, L.; Spinelli, L. Time domain functional NIRS imaging for human brain mapping. *Neuroimage* **2014**, *85*, 28–50. [CrossRef]
11. Konugolu Venkata Sekar, S.; Lanka, P.; Farina, A.; Dalla Mora, A.; Andersson-Engels, S.; Taroni, P.; Pifferi, A. Broadband Time Domain Diffuse Optical Reflectance Spectroscopy: A Review of Systems, Methods, and Applications. *Appl. Sci.* **2019**, *9*, 5465. [CrossRef]
12. Hoshi, Y.; Yamada, Y. Overview of diffuse optical tomography and its clinical applications. *J. Biomed. Opt.* **2016**, *21*, 091312. [CrossRef]
13. Durduran, T.; Choe, R.; Baker, W.B.; Yodh, A.G. Diffuse optics for tissue monitoring and tomography. *Rep. Prog. Phys.* **2010**, *73*, 076701. [CrossRef]
14. Labruyère, A.; Tonello, A.; Couderc, V.; Huss, G.; Leproux, P. Compact supercontinuum sources and their biomedical applications. *Opt. Fiber Technol.* **2012**, *18*, 375–378. [CrossRef]
15. Alfano, R.R.; Shapiro, S.L. Emission in the Region 4000 to 7000 A Via Four-Photon Coupling in Glass. *Phys. Rev. Lett.* **1970**, *24*, 584–587. [CrossRef]
16. Alfano, R.R.; Shapiro, S.L. Observation of Self-Phase Modulation and Small-Scale Filaments in Crystals and Glasses. *Phys. Rev. Lett.* **1970**, *24*, 592–594. [CrossRef]
17. Granzow, N. Supercontinuum white light lasers: A review on technology and applications. In Proceedings of the Joint TC1—TC2 International Symposium on Photonics and Education in Measurement Science, Jena, Germany, 17–19 September 2019; Volume 11144, p. 1114408.
18. Bloembergen, N. Nonlinear optics: Past, present, and future. *IEEE J. Sel. Top. Quantum Electron.* **2000**, *6*, 876–880. [CrossRef]
19. Agrawal, G.P. Nonlinear fiber optics: Its history and recent progress [Invited]. *J. Opt. Soc. Am. B* **2011**, *28*, A1–A10. [CrossRef]
20. Knight, J.C.; Birks, T.A.; Russell, P.S.J.; Atkin, D.M. All-silica single-mode optical fiber with photonic crystal cladding. *Opt. Lett.* **1996**, *21*, 1547–1549. [CrossRef] [PubMed]
21. Tu, H.; Boppart, S.A. Coherent fiber supercontinuum for biophotonics. *Laser Photonics Rev.* **2013**, *7*, 628–645. [CrossRef]
22. Pifferi, A.; Contini, D.; Mora, A.D.; Farina, A.; Spinelli, L.; Torricelli, A. New frontiers in time-domain diffuse optics, a review. *J. Biomed. Opt.* **2016**, *21*, 091310. [CrossRef] [PubMed]

23. Konugolu Venkata Sekar, S.; Dalla Mora, A.; Bargigia, I.; Martinenghi, E.; Lindner, C.; Farzam, P.; Pagliazzi, M.; Durduran, T.; Taroni, P.; Pifferi, A.; et al. Broadband (600–1350 nm) Time-Resolved Diffuse Optical Spectrometer for Clinical Use. *IEEE J. Sel. Top. Quantum Electron.* **2016**, *22*, 406–414. [CrossRef]
24. Lange, F.; Dunne, L.; Hale, L.; Tachtsidis, I. MAESTROS: A Multiwavelength Time-Domain NIRS System to Monitor Changes in Oxygenation and Oxidation State of Cytochrome-C-Oxidase. *IEEE J. Sel. Top. Quantum Electron.* **2018**, *25*. [CrossRef] [PubMed]
25. Giannoni, L.; Lange, F.; Sajic, M.; Smith, K.J.; Tachtsidis, I. A hyperspectral imaging system for mapping haemoglobin and cytochrome-c-oxidase concentration changes in the exposed cerebral cortex. *IEEE J. Sel. Top. Quantum Electron.* **2021**, *27*. [CrossRef] [PubMed]
26. Jiang, J.; Mata, A.D.C.; Lindner, S.; Charbon, E.; Wolf, M.; Kalyanov, A. Dynamic time domain near-infrared optical tomography based on a SPAD camera. *Biomed. Opt. Express* **2020**, *11*, 5470. [CrossRef]
27. Jiang, J.; Mata, A.D.C.; Lindner, S.; Zhang, C.; Charbon, E.; Wolf, M.; Kalyanov, A. Image reconstruction for novel time domain near infrared optical tomography: Towards clinical applications. *Biomed. Opt. Express* **2020**, *11*, 4723. [CrossRef] [PubMed]
28. Cooper, R.J.; Magee, E.; Everdell, N.; Magazov, S.; Varela, M.; Airantzis, D.; Gibson, A.P.; Hebden, J.C. MONSTIR II: A 32-channel, multispectral, time-resolved optical tomography system for neonatal brain imaging. *Rev. Sci. Instrum.* **2014**, *85*. [CrossRef] [PubMed]
29. Andersson-Engels, S.; Berg, R.; Persson, A.; Svanberg, S. Multispectral tissue characterization with time-resolved detection of diffusely scattered white light. *Opt. Lett.* **1993**, *18*, 1697. [CrossRef]
30. af Klinteberg, C.; Berg, R.; Lindquist, C.; Andersson-Engels, S.; Svanberg, S. Diffusely scattered femtosecond white-light examination of breast tissue in vitro and in vivo. *Photon Propag. Tissues* **1995**, *2626*, 149–157.
31. Jarlman, O.; Berg, R.; Andersson-Engels, S.; Svanberg, S.; Pettersson, H. Time-resolved white light transillumination for optical imaging. *Acta Radiol.* **1997**, *38*, 185–189. [CrossRef]
32. Abrahamsson, C.; Svensson, T.; Svanberg, S.; Andersson-Engels, S.; Johansson, J.; Folestad, S. Time and wavelength resolved spectroscopy of turbid media using light continuum generated in a crystal fiber. *Opt. Express* **2004**, *12*, 4103–4112. [CrossRef]
33. Pifferi, A.; Torricelli, A.; Taroni, P.; Comelli, D.; Bassi, A.; Cubeddu, R. Fully automated time domain spectrometer for the absorption and scattering characterization of diffusive media. *Rev. Sci. Instrum.* **2007**, *78*, 053103. [CrossRef] [PubMed]
34. Taroni, P.; Pifferi, A.; Torricelli, A.; Comelli, D.; Cubeddu, R. In vivo absorption and scattering spectroscopy of biological tissues. *Photochem. Photobiol. Sci.* **2003**, *2*, 124–129. [CrossRef]
35. Pifferi, A.; Torricelli, A.; Taroni, P.; Bassi, A.; Chikoidze, E.; Giambattistelli, E.; Cubeddu, R. Optical biopsy of bone tissue: A step toward the diagnosis of bone pathologies. *J. Biomed. Opt.* **2004**, *9*, 474. [CrossRef] [PubMed]
36. Cubeddu, R.; Pifferi, A.; Taroni, P.; Torricelli, A.; Valentini, G. Noninvasive absorption and scattering spectroscopy of bulk diffusive media: An application to the optical characterization of human breast. *Appl. Phys. Lett.* **1999**, *74*, 874–876. [CrossRef]
37. Taroni, P.; Pifferi, A.; Cubeddu, R.; Torricelli, A.; Comelli, D. Absorption of collagen: Effects on the estimate of breast composition and related diagnostic implications. *J. Biomed. Opt.* **2007**, *12*, 014021. [CrossRef]
38. Bassi, A.; Farina, A.; D'Andrea, C.; Pifferi, A.; Valentini, G.; Cubeddu, R. Portable, large-bandwidth time-resolved system for diffuse optical spectroscopy. *Opt. Express* **2007**, *15*, 14482. [CrossRef]
39. Taroni, P.; Bassi, A.; Comelli, D.; Farina, A.; Cubeddu, R.; Pifferi, A. Diffuse optical spectroscopy of breast tissue extended to 1100 nm. *J. Biomed. Opt.* **2009**, *14*, 054030. [CrossRef] [PubMed]
40. Farina, A.; Bassi, A.; Pifferi, A.; Taroni, P.; Comelli, D.; Spinelli, L.; Cubeddu, R. Bandpass Effects in Time-Resolved Diffuse Spectroscopy. *Appl. Spectrosc.* **2009**, *63*, 48–56. [CrossRef]
41. Farina, A.; Bargigia, I.; Taroni, P.; Pifferi, A. Note: Comparison between a prism-based and an acousto-optic tunable filter-based spectrometer for diffusive media. *Rev. Sci. Instrum.* **2013**, *84*. [CrossRef]
42. Svensson, T.; Alerstam, E.; Khoptyar, D.; Johansson, J.; Folestad, S.; Andersson-Engels, S. Near-infrared photon time-of-flight spectroscopy of turbid materials up to 1400 nm. *Rev. Sci. Instrum.* **2009**, *80*, 45–48. [CrossRef]
43. Bargigia, I.; Tosi, A.; Farina, A.; Bassi, A.; Taroni, P.; Bahgat Shehata, A.; Della Frera, A.; Dalla Mora, A.; Zappa, F.; Cubeddu, R.; et al. Optical Spectroscopy up to 1700 nm: A Time-Resolved Approach Combined with an InGaAs/InP Single-Photon Avalanche Diode. In Proceedings of the Biomedical Optics and 3-D Imaging 2012, Miami, FL, USA, 28 April–2 May 2012; p. JM3A.16.
44. Bargigia, I.; Tosi, A.; Bahgat Shehata, A.; Della Frera, A.; Farina, A.; Bassi, A.; Taroni, P.; Dalla Mora, A.; Zappa, F.; Cubeddu, R.; et al. Time-resolved diffuse optical spectroscopy up to 1700 nm by means of a time-gated InGaAs/InP single-photon avalanche diode. *Appl. Spectrosc.* **2012**, *66*, 944–950. [CrossRef]
45. Bargigia, I.; Tosi, A.; Bahgat Shehata, A.; Della Frera, A.; Farina, A.; Bassi, A.; Taroni, P.; Dalla Mora, A.; Zappa, F.; Cubeddu, R.; et al. In-vivo optical spectroscopy in the time-domain beyond 1100 nm. In Proceedings of the Optics InfoBase Conference Papers, Munich, Germany, 12–16 May 2013; Taroni, P., Dehghani, H., Eds.; Optical Society of America: Washington, DC, USA, 2013; p. 879902.
46. Sekar, S.K.V.; Bargigia, I.; Mora, A.D.; Taroni, P.; Ruggeri, A.; Tosi, A.; Pifferi, A.; Farina, A. Diffuse optical characterization of collagen absorption from 500 to 1700 nm. *J. Biomed. Opt.* **2017**, *22*, 015006. [CrossRef] [PubMed]
47. Konugolu Venkata Sekar, S.; Farina, A.; Martinenghi, E.; Dalla Mora, A.; Taroni, P.; Pifferi, A.; Negredo, E.; Puig, J.; Escrig, R.; Rosales, Q.; et al. Time-resolved diffused optical characterization of key tissue constituents of human bony prominence locations. In Proceedings of the European Conference on Biomedical Optics, Munich, Germany, 21–25 June 2015; Volume 9538, pp. 95380X–95380X–5.

48. Konugolu Venkata Sekar, S.; Pagliazzi, M.; Negredo, E.; Martelli, F.; Farina, A.; Dalla Mora, A.; Lindner, C.; Farzam, P.; Pérez-Álvarez, N.; Puig, J.; et al. In Vivo, non-invasive characterization of human bone by hybrid broadband (600–1200 nm) diffuse optical and correlation spectroscopies. *PLoS ONE* **2016**, *11*, e0168426. [CrossRef]
49. Sekar, S.K.V.; Mora, A.D.; Martinenghi, E.; Taroni, P.; Pifferi, A.; Farina, A.; Puig, J.; Negredo, E.; Lindner, C.; Pagliazzi, M.; et al. In vivo Time domain Broadband (600–1200 nm) Diffuse Optical Characterization of Human Bone. In Proceedings of the Optical Tomography and Spectroscopy 2016, Fort Lauderdale, FL, USA, 25–28 April 2016; p. JTu3A.32.
50. Konugolu Venkata Sekar, S.; Farina, A.; Dalla Mora, A.; Lindner, C.; Pagliazzi, M.; Mora, M.; Aranda, G.; Dehghani, H.; Durduran, T.; Taroni, P.; et al. Broadband (550–1350 nm) diffuse optical characterization of thyroid chromophores. *Sci. Rep.* **2018**, *8*, 1–8. [CrossRef]
51. Lanka, P.; Segala, A.; Farina, A.; Konugolu Venkata Sekar, S.; Nisoli, E.; Valerio, A.; Taroni, P.; Cubeddu, R.; Pifferi, A. Non-invasive investigation of adipose tissue by time domain diffuse optical spectroscopy. *Biomed. Opt. Express* **2020**, *11*, 2779. [CrossRef] [PubMed]
52. Taroni, P.; Bassi, A.; Farina, A.; Cubeddu, R.; Pifferi, A. Role of Collagen Scattering for in vivo Tissue Characterization. In Proceedings of the Biomedical Optics 2010, Miami, FL, USA, 11–14 April 2010; p. BTuD107.
53. Konugolu Venkata Sekar, S.; Beh, J.S.; Farina, A.; Dalla Mora, A.; Pifferi, A.; Taroni, P. Broadband diffuse optical characterization of elastin for biomedical applications. *Biophys. Chem.* **2017**, *229*, 130–134. [CrossRef] [PubMed]
54. Ferocino, E.; Di Sciacca, G.; Di Sieno, L.; Dalla Mora, A.; Pifferi, A.; Arridge, S.R.; Martelli, F.; Taroni, P.; Farina, A. Multi-wavelength time domain diffuse optical tomography for breast cancer: Initial results on silicone phantoms. In Proceedings of the SPIE BiOS, San Francisco, CA, USA, 2–7 February 2019; p. 59.
55. Taroni, P.; Pifferi, A.; Quarto, G.; Farina, A.; Ieva, F.; Paganoni, A.M.; Abbate, F.; Cassano, E.; Cubeddu, R. Time domain diffuse optical spectroscopy: In vivo quantification of collagen in breast tissue. In Proceedings of the Optical Methods for Inspection, Characterization, and Imaging of Biomaterials II, Munich, Germany, 21–25 June 2015; Volume 9529, p. 952910.
56. Lanka, P.; Joseph, F.K.; Kruit, H.; Konugolu, S.; Sekar, V.; Farina, A.; Cubeddu, R.; Manohar, S.; Pifferi, A. Time domain diffuse optical spectroscopy for the monitoring of thermal treatment in biological tissue. In Proceedings of the Optical Tomography and Spectroscopy 2020, Washington, DC, USA, 20–23 April 2020; pp. 1–2.
57. Kalloor Joseph, F.; Lanka, P.; Kruit, H.; Konugolu Venkata Sekar, S.; Farina, A.; Cubeddu, R.; Manohar, S.; Pifferi, A. Key features in the optical properties of tissue during and after radiofrequency ablation. In Proceedings of the SPIE BiOS, San Francisco, CA, USA, 1–6 February 2020; p. 16.
58. Bassi, A.; Spinelli, L.; D'Andrea, C.; Giusto, A.; Swartling, J.; Pifferi, A.; Torricelli, A.; Cubeddu, R. Feasibility of white-light time-resolved optical mammography. *J. Biomed. Opt.* **2006**, *11*, 054035. [CrossRef]
59. Ferrari, M.; Mottola, L.; Quaresima, V. Principles, techniques, and limitations of near infrared spectroscopy. *Can. J. Appl. Physiol.* **2004**, *29*, 463–487. [CrossRef]
60. Bassi, A.; Swartling, J.; D'Andrea, C.; Pifferi, A.; Torricelli, A.; Cubeddu, R. Time-resolved spectrophotometer for turbid media based on supercontinuum generation in a photonic crystal fiber. *Opt. Lett.* **2004**, *29*, 2405. [CrossRef]
61. Swartling, J.; Bassi, A.; D'Andrea, C.; Pifferi, A.; Torricelli, A.; Cubeddu, R. Dynamic time-resolved diffuse spectroscopy based on supercontinuum light pulses. *Appl. Opt.* **2005**, *44*, 4684. [CrossRef] [PubMed]
62. Gerega, A.; Milej, D.; Weigl, W.; Kacprzak, M.; Liebert, A. Multiwavelength time-resolved near-infrared spectroscopy of the adult head: Assessment of intracerebral and extracerebral absorption changes. *Biomed. Opt. Express* **2018**, *9*, 2974. [CrossRef]
63. Gerega, A.; Milej, D.; Weigl, W.; Zolek, N.; Sawosz, P.; Maniewski, R.; Liebert, A. Multi-wavelength time-resolved measurements of diffuse reflectance: Phantom study with dynamic inflow of ICG. In Proceedings of the Biomedical Optics 2012, Miami, FL, USA, 28 April–2 May 2012; p. JM3A.31.
64. Sudakou, A.; Lange, F.; Isler, H.; Gerega, A.; Ostojic, D.; Sawosz, P.; Tachtsidis, I.; Wolf, M.; Liebert, A. Multi-wavelength time-resolved NIRS measurements for estimation of absolute concentration of chromophores: Blood phantom study. In Proceedings of the Diffuse Optical Spectroscopy and Imaging VII, Munich, Germany, 23–25 June 2019; Dehghani, H., Wabnitz, H., Eds.; SPIE: Washington, DC, USA, 2019; Volume 1107422, p. 72.
65. He, L.; Baker, W.B.; Busch, D.R.; Jiang, J.Y.; Lawrence, K.S.; Kofke, W.A.; Yodh, A.G.; He, L.; Baker, W.B.; Milej, D.; et al. Noninvasive continuous optical monitoring of absolute cerebral blood flow in critically ill adults. *Neurophotonics* **2018**, *5*, 1.
66. Durduran, T.; Yodh, A.G. Diffuse correlation spectroscopy for non-invasive, micro-vascular cerebral blood flow measurement. *Neuroimage* **2014**, *85*, 5163. [CrossRef] [PubMed]
67. Selb, J.; Zimmermann, B.B.; Martino, M.; Ogden, T.; Boas, D.A. Functional brain imaging with a supercontinuum time-domain NIRS system. In Proceedings of the Optical Tomography and Spectroscopy of Tissue X, San Francisco, CA, USA, 5–7 February 2013; Volume 8578, p. 857807.
68. Selb, J.; Joseph, D.K.; Boas, D. Time-gated optical system for depth-resolved functional brain imaging. *J. Biomed. Opt.* **2006**, *11*, 44008. [CrossRef]
69. Lange, F.; Peyrin, F.; Montcel, B. Broadband time-resolved multi-channel functional near-infrared spectroscopy system to monitor in vivo physiological changes of human brain activity. *Appl. Opt.* **2018**, *57*, 6417. [CrossRef]
70. Lange, F.; Peyrin, F.; Montcel, B. A hyperspectral time resolved DOT system to monitor physiological changes of the human brain activity. In Proceedings of the Advanced Microscopy Techniques IV and Neurophotonics II, Munich, Germany, 21–25 June 2015; OSA: Washington, DC, USA, 2015; p. 95360R.

71. Lange, F.; Dunne, L.; Tachtsidis, I. Evaluation of Haemoglobin and Cytochrome Responses During Forearm Ischaemia Using Multi-wavelength Time Domain NIRS. In *Oxygen Transport to Tissue XXXIX*; Advances in Experimental Medicine and Biology; Halpern, H.J., LaManna, J.C., Harrison, D.K., Epel, B., Eds.; Springer International Publishing: Cham, Switzerland, 2017; Volume 977, pp. 67–72. ISBN 978-3-319-55229-3.
72. Lange, F.; Tachtsidis, I. Short and mid-term reproducibility analysis of cerebral tissue saturation measured by time domain-NIRS. In Proceedings of the European Conference on Biomedical Optics, Munich, Germany, 23–25 June 2019; Volume 11074.
73. Mazurenka, M.; Jelzow, A.; Wabnitz, H.; Contini, D.; Spinelli, L.; Pifferi, A.; Cubeddu, R.; Mora, A.D.; Tosi, A.; Zappa, F.; et al. Non-contact time-resolved diffuse reflectance imaging at null source-detector separation. *Opt. Express* **2011**, *20*, 283. [CrossRef]
74. Wabnitz, H.; Mazurenka, M.; Di Sieno, L.; Contini, D.; Dalla Mora, A.; Farina, A.; Hoshi, Y.; Kirilina, E.; Macdonald, R.; Pifferi, A. Non-contact time-domain imaging of functional brain activation and heterogeneity of superficial signals. In Proceedings of the Diffuse Optical Spectroscopy and Imaging VI, Munich, Germany, 25–29 June 2017; Dehghani, H., Wabnitz, H., Eds.; SPIE: Washington, DC, USA, 2017; Volume 10412, p. 104120J.
75. Mazurenka, M.; Di Sieno, L.; Boso, G.; Contini, D.; Pifferi, A.; Mora, A.D.; Tosi, A.; Wabnitz, H.; Macdonald, R. Non-contact in vivo diffuse optical imaging using a time-gated scanning system. *Biomed. Opt. Express* **2013**, *4*, 2257. [CrossRef]
76. Di Sieno, L.; Wabnitz, H.; Pifferi, A.; Mazurenka, M.; Hoshi, Y.; Dalla Mora, A.; Contini, D.; Boso, G.; Becker, W.; Martelli, F.; et al. Characterization of a time-resolved non-contact scanning diffuse optical imaging system exploiting fast-gated single-photon avalanche diode detection. *Rev. Sci. Instrum.* **2016**, *87*. [CrossRef]
77. Torricelli, A.; Pifferi, A.; Spinelli, L.; Cubeddu, R.; Martelli, F.; Del Bianco, S.; Zaccanti, G. Time-Resolved Reflectance at Null Source-Detector Separation: Improving Contrast and Resolution in Diffuse Optical Imaging. *Phys. Rev. Lett.* **2005**, *95*, 078101. [CrossRef]
78. Dalla Mora, A.; Tosi, A.; Zappa, F.; Cova, S.; Contini, D.; Pifferi, A.; Spinelli, L.; Torricelli, A.; Cubeddu, R. Fast-Gated Single-Photon Avalanche Diode for Wide Dynamic Range Near Infrared Spectroscopy. *IEEE J. Sel. Top. Quantum Electron.* **2010**, *16*, 1023–1030. [CrossRef]
79. Contini, D.; Dalla Mora, A.; Spinelli, L.; Farina, A.; Torricelli, A.; Cubeddu, R.; Martelli, F.; Zaccanti, G.; Tosi, A.; Boso, G.; et al. Effects of time-gated detection in diffuse optical imaging at short source-detector separation. *J. Phys. D Appl. Phys.* **2015**, *48*, 045401. [CrossRef]
80. Mottin, S.; Montcel, B.; de Chatellus, H.G.; Ramstein, S.; Vignal, C.; Mathevon, N. Functional White-Laser Imaging to Study Brain Oxygen Uncoupling/Recoupling in Songbirds. *J. Cereb. Blood Flow Metab.* **2011**, *31*, 393–400. [CrossRef]
81. Ramstein, S.; Vignal, C.; Mathevon, N.; Mottin, S. In vivo and noninvasive measurement of a songbird head's optical properties. *Appl. Opt.* **2005**, *44*, 6197. [CrossRef]
82. Torabzadeh, M.; Stockton, P.; Kennedy, G.T.; Saager, R.B.; Durkin, A.J.; Bartels, R.A.; Tromberg, B.J. Hyperspectral imaging in the spatial frequency domain with a supercontinuum source. *J. Biomed. Opt.* **2019**, *24*, 1. [CrossRef] [PubMed]
83. Farina, A.; Lepore, M.; Di Sieno, L.; Dalla Mora, A.; Ducros, N.; Pifferi, A.; Valentini, G.; Arridge, S.; D'Andrea, C. Diffuse optical tomography by using time-resolved single pixel camera. In Proceedings of the SPIE BiOS, San Francisco, CA, USA, 7–12 February 2015; Tromberg, B.J., Yodh, A.G., Sevick-Muraca, E.M., Alfano, R.R., Eds.; International Society for Optics and Photonics: Bellingham, WA, USA, 2015; p. 93191K.
84. Pian, Q.; Yao, R.; Intes, X. Hyperspectral wide-field time domain single-pixel diffuse optical tomography platform. *Biomed. Opt. Express* **2018**, *9*, 6258. [CrossRef]
85. Valim, N.; Brock, J.; Niedre, M. Experimental measurement of time-dependent photon scatter for diffuse optical tomography. *J. Biomed. Opt.* **2010**, *15*, 065006. [CrossRef]
86. Zouaoui, J.; Di Sieno, L.; Hervé, L.; Pifferi, A.; Farina, A.; Mora, A.D.; Derouard, J.; Dinten, J.-M. Chromophore decomposition in multispectral time-resolved diffuse optical tomography. *Biomed. Opt. Express* **2017**, *8*, 4772. [CrossRef]
87. Di Sieno, L.; Bettega, G.; Berger, M.; Hamou, C.; Aribert, M.; Mora, A.D.; Puszka, A.; Grateau, H.; Contini, D.; Hervé, L.; et al. Toward noninvasive assessment of flap viability with time-resolved diffuse optical tomography: A preclinical test on rats. *J. Biomed. Opt.* **2016**, *21*, 025004. [CrossRef]
88. Dempsey, L.A.; Cooper, R.J.; Powell, S.; Edwards, A.; Lee, C.-W.; Brigadoi, S.; Everdell, N.; Arridge, S.; Gibson, A.P.; Austin, T.; et al. Whole-head functional brain imaging of neonates at cot-side using time-resolved diffuse optical tomography. In Proceedings of the Diffuse Optical Imaging V, Munich, Germany, 21–25 June 2015; Volume 9538, pp. 1–10.
89. Dempsey, L.A. Development and Application of Diffuse Optical Tomography Systems for Diagnosis and Assessment of Perinatal Brain Injury. Ph.D. Thesis, University College London, London, UK, 2018.
90. Jiang, J.; Ahnen, L.; Kalyanov, A.; Lindner, S.; Wolf, M.; Majos, S.S. A New Method Based on Graphics Processing Units for Fast Near-Infrared Optical Tomography. *Adv. Exp. Med. Biol.* **2017**, *977*, 191–197.
91. Arnesano, C.; Santoro, Y.; Gratton, E. Digital parallel frequency-domain spectroscopy for tissue imaging. *J. Biomed. Opt.* **2012**, *17*, 0960141. [CrossRef] [PubMed]
92. Pifferi, A.; Torricelli, A.; Bassi, A.; Taroni, P.; Cubeddu, R.; Wabnitz, H.; Grosenick, D.; Möller, M.; Macdonald, R.; Swartling, J.; et al. Performance assessment of photon migration instruments: The MEDPHOT protocol. *Appl. Opt.* **2005**, *44*, 2104–2114. [CrossRef] [PubMed]

93. Wabnitz, H.; Jelzow, A.; Mazurenka, M.; Steinkellner, O.; Macdonald, R.; Milej, D.; Zolek, N.; Kacprzak, M.; Sawosz, P.; Maniewski, R.; et al. Performance assessment of time-domain optical brain imagers, part 1: Basic instrumental performance protocol. *J. Biomed. Opt.* **2014**, *19*, 86010. [CrossRef] [PubMed]
94. Wabnitz, H.; Jelzow, A.; Mazurenka, M.; Steinkellner, O.; Macdonald, R.; Milej, D.; Zolek, N.; Kacprzak, M.; Sawosz, P.; Maniewski, R.; et al. Performance assessment of time-domain optical brain imagers, part 2: nEUROPt protocol. *J. Biomed. Opt.* **2014**, *19*, 086012. [CrossRef]
95. Quarto, G.; Pifferi, A.; Bargigia, I.; Farina, A.; Cubeddu, R.; Taroni, P. Recipes to make organic phantoms for diffusive optical spectroscopy. *Appl. Opt.* **2013**, *52*, 2494–2502. [CrossRef]
96. Wang, L.; Sharma, S.; Aernouts, B.; Ramon, H.; Saeys, W. Supercontinuum laser based double-integrating-sphere system for measuring optical properties of highly dense turbid media in the 1300–2350 nm region with high sensitivity. In Proceedings of the SPIE Photonics Europe, Brussels, Belgium, 16–19 April 2012; Volume 8427, p. 84273B.
97. Spinelli, L.; Botwicz, M.; Zolek, N.; Kacprzak, M.; Milej, D.; Liebert, A.; Weigel, U.; Durduran, T.; Foschum, F.; Kienle, A.; et al. Inter-Laboratory Comparison of Optical Properties Performed on Intralipid and India Ink. In Proceedings of the Biomedical Optics and 3-D Imaging, Miami, FL, USA, 28 April–2 May 2012; OSA: Washington, DC, USA, 2012; p. BW1A.6.
98. Aernouts, B.; Zamora-Rojas, E.; Van Beers, R.; Watté, R.; Wang, L.; Tsuta, M.; Lammertyn, J.; Saeys, W. Supercontinuum laser based optical characterization of Intralipid®phantoms in the 500–2250 nm range. *Opt. Express* **2013**, *21*, 32450. [CrossRef]
99. Aernouts, B.; Van Beers, R.; Watté, R.; Lammertyn, J.; Saeys, W. Dependent scattering in Intralipid®phantoms in the 600–1850 nm range. *Opt. Express* **2014**, *22*, 6086. [CrossRef]
100. Spinelli, L.; Botwicz, M.; Zolek, N.; Kacprzak, M.; Milej, D.; Sawosz, P.; Liebert, A.; Weigel, U.; Durduran, T.; Foschum, F.; et al. Determination of reference values for optical properties of liquid phantoms based on Intralipid and India ink. *Biomed. Opt. Express* **2014**, *5*, 2037. [CrossRef]
101. Bouchard, J.-P.; Veilleux, I.; Jedidi, R.; Noiseux, I.; Fortin, M.; Mermut, O. Reference optical phantoms for diffuse optical spectroscopy. Part 1—Error analysis of a time resolved transmittance characterization method. *Opt. Express* **2010**, *18*, 11495–11507. [CrossRef]
102. Martelli, F.; Di Ninni, P.; Zaccanti, G.; Contini, D.; Spinelli, L.; Torricelli, A.; Cubeddu, R.; Wabnitz, H.; Mazurenka, M.; Macdonald, R.; et al. Phantoms for diffuse optical imaging based on totally absorbing objects, part 2: Experimental implementation. *J. Biomed. Opt.* **2014**, *19*, 076011. [CrossRef]
103. Pifferi, A.; Torricelli, A.; Cubeddu, R.; Quarto, G.; Re, R.; Sekar, S.K.V.; Spinelli, L.; Farina, A.; Martelli, F.; Wabnitz, H. Mechanically switchable solid inhomogeneous phantom for performance tests in diffuse imaging and spectroscopy. *J. Biomed. Opt.* **2015**, *20*, 121304. [CrossRef] [PubMed]
104. Wabnitz, H.; Taubert, D.R.; Funane, T.; Kiguchi, M.; Eda, H.; Pifferi, A.; Torricelli, A.; Macdonald, R. Characterization of homogeneous tissue phantoms for performance tests in diffuse optics. In Proceedings of the SPIE BiOS, San Francisco, CA, USA, 13–18 February 2016; Volume 9700, p. 970004.
105. Xu, R.X.; Allen, D.W.; Huang, J.; Gnyawali, S.; Melvin, J.; Elgharably, H.; Gordillo, G.; Huang, K.; Bergdall, V.; Litorja, M.; et al. Developing digital tissue phantoms for hyperspectral imaging of ischemic wounds. *Biomed. Opt. Express* **2012**, *3*, 1433. [CrossRef]
106. Wabnitz, H.; Hwang, J.; Yang, L.; Macdonald, R. Digital phantom for time-domain near-infrared spectroscopy of tissue: Concept and proof-of-principle experiments. In Proceedings of the SPIE BiOS, San Francisco, CA, USA, 2–7 February 2019; p. 20.
107. Spinelli, L.; Rizzolo, A.; Vanoli, M.; Grassi, M.; Zerbini, P.E.; Pimentel, R.; Torricelli, A. Optical properties of pulp and skin in Brazilian mangoes in the 540–900 nm spectral range: Implication for non-destructive maturity assessment by time-resolved reflectance spectroscopy. In Proceedings of the International Conference of Agricultural Engineering, CIGR-AgEng2012, Valencia, Spain, 8–12 July 2012; p. C–2096.
108. Amendola, C.; Pirovano, I.; Lacerenza, M.; Contini, D.; Spinelli, L.; Cubeddu, R.; Torricelli, A.; Re, R. Use of 3D printed PLA for diffuse optics. In Proceedings of the Biophotonics Congress: Biomedical Optics 2020 (Translational, Microscopy, OCT, OTS, BRAIN), Washington, DC, USA, 20–23 April 2020; pp. 32–33.
109. Dalla Mora, A.; Martinenghi, E.; Contini, D.; Tosi, A.; Boso, G.; Durduran, T.; Arridge, S.; Martelli, F.; Farina, A.; Torricelli, A.; et al. Fast silicon photomultiplier improves signal harvesting and reduces complexity in time-domain diffuse optics. *Opt. Express* **2015**, *23*, 13937–13946. [CrossRef]
110. Martinenghi, E.; Dalla Mora, A.; Contini, D.; Farina, A.; Villa, F.; Torricelli, A.; Pifferi, A. Spectrally Resolved Single-Photon Timing of Silicon Photomultipliers for Time-Domain Diffuse Spectroscopy. *IEEE Photonics J.* **2015**, *7*, 1–12. [CrossRef]
111. Martinenghi, E.; Di Sieno, L.; Contini, D.; Sanzaro, M.; Pifferi, A.; Dalla Mora, A. Time-resolved single-photon detection module based on silicon photomultiplier: A novel building block for time-correlated measurement systems. *Rev. Sci. Instrum.* **2016**, *87*. [CrossRef] [PubMed]
112. Di Sieno, L.; Boetti, N.G.; Mora, A.D.; Pugliese, D.; Farina, A.; Konugolu Venkata Sekar, S.; Ceci-Ginistrelli, E.; Janner, D.; Pifferi, A.; Milanese, D. Towards the use of bioresorbable fibers in time-domain diffuse optics. *J. Biophotonics* **2017**, *11*, 1–12. [CrossRef] [PubMed]
113. Mora, A.D.; Di Sieno, L.; Venkata Sekar, S.K.; Farina, A.; Contini, D.; Boetti, N.G.; Milanese, D.; Nissinen, J.; Pifferi, A. Novel technologies for time-domain diffuse optics: Miniaturized wearable devices and bioresorbable optical fibers. In Proceedings of the Biophotonics Congress: Biomedical Optics Congress 2018 (Microscopy/Translational/Brain/OTS), Hollywood, FL, USA, 3–6 April 2018; p. F90-O.

114. D'Andrea, C.; Spinelli, L.; Bassi, A.; Giusto, A.; Contini, D.; Swartling, J.; Torricelli, A.; Cubeddu, R. Time-resolved spectrally constrained method for the quantification of chromophore concentrations and scattering parameters in diffusing media. *Opt. Express* **2006**, *14*, 1888. [CrossRef] [PubMed]
115. Giusto, A.; D'Andrea, C.; Spinelli, L.; Contini, D.; Torricelli, A.; Martelli, F.; Zaccanti, G.; Cubeddu, R. Monitoring absorption changes in a layered diffusive medium by white-light time-resolved reflectance spectroscopy. *IEEE Trans. Instrum. Meas.* **2010**, *59*, 1925–1932. [CrossRef]
116. Pifferi, A.; Bassi, A.; Spinelli, L.; Cubeddu, R.; Taroni, P. Time-Resolved Broadband Diffuse Spectroscopy Using a Differential Absorption Approach. In Proceedings of the Biomedical Optics and 3-D Imaging, Miami, FL, USA, 11–14 April 2010; p. BSuD45; Volume 64, p. BSuD45.
117. Yang, L.; Wabnitz, H.; Gladytz, T.; Macdonald, R.; Grosenick, D. Spatially-enhanced time-domain NIRS for accurate determination of tissue optical properties. *Opt. Express* **2019**, *27*, 26415. [CrossRef] [PubMed]
118. Yang, L.; Lanka, P.; Wabnitz, H.; Cubeddu, R.; Gladytz, T.; Konugolu Venkata Sekar, S.; Grosenick, D.; Pifferi, A.; Macdonald, R. Spatially-enhanced time-domain NIRS for determination of optical properties in layered structures. In Proceedings of the European Conference on Biomedical Optics, Munich, Germany, 23–25 June 2019; p. 9.
119. Yang, L.; Wabnitz, H.; Gladytz, T.; Sudakou, A.; Macdonald, R.; Grosenick, D. Space-enhanced time-domain diffuse optics for determination of tissue optical properties in two-layered structures. *Biomed. Opt. Express* **2020**, *11*, 6570. [CrossRef]
120. Wojtkiewicz, S.; Gerega, A.; Zanoletti, M.; Sudakou, A.; Contini, D.; Liebert, A.; Durduran, T.; Dehghani, H. Self-calibrating time-resolved near infrared spectroscopy. *Biomed. Opt. Express* **2019**, *10*, 2657. [CrossRef]
121. Kovacsova, Z.; Bale, G.; Mitra, S.; Lange, F.; Tachtsidis, I. Absolute quantification of cerebral tissue oxygen saturation with multidistance broadband NIRS in newborn brain. *Biomed. Opt. Express* **2021**, *12*, 907. [CrossRef]
122. Wabnitz, H.; Contini, D.; Spinelli, L.; Torricelli, A.; Liebert, A. Depth-selective analysis in time-domain optical brain imaging: Moments vs. time windows. *Biomed. Opt. Express* **2020**, *11*, 4224–4243. [CrossRef] [PubMed]
123. Sudakou, A.; Yang, L.; Wabnitz, H.; Wojtkiewicz, S.; Liebert, A. Performance of measurands in time-domain optical brain imaging: Depth selectivity versus contrast-to-noise ratio. *Biomed. Opt. Express* **2020**, *11*, 4348–4365. [CrossRef]
124. Lanka, P.; Yang, L.; Orive-Miguel, D.; Veesa, J.D.; Tagliabue, S.; Sudakou, A.; Samaei, S.; Forcione, M.; Kovacsova, Z.; Behera, A.; et al. The BITMAP exercise: A multi-laboratory performance assessment campaign of diffuse optical instrumentation. In Proceedings of the Diffuse Optical Spectroscopy and Imaging VII, Munich, Germany, 23–25 June 2019; Dehghani, H., Wabnitz, H., Eds.; SPIE: Washington, DC, USA; p. 44.
125. Orive-Miguel, D.; Lanka, P.; Yang, L.; Tagliabue, S.; Sudakou, A.; Samaei, S.; Veesa, J.D.; Forcione, M.; Kovacsova, Z.; Behera, A.; et al. The BitMap dataset: An open dataset on performance assessment of diffuse optics instruments. In Proceedings of the European Conference on Biomedical Optics 2019, Munich, Germany, 23–25 June 2019; p. 45.
126. Farina, A.; Pifferi, A.; Torricelli, A.; Bargigia, I.; Spinelli, L.; Cubeddu, R.; Foschum, F.; Jäger, M.; Simon, E.; Fugger, O.; et al. Multi-center study of the optical properties of the human head. In Proceedings of the Biomedical Optics 2014, Miami, FL, USA, 26–30 April 2014; Volume 6, p. BS3A.9.
127. Sordillo, L.A.; Lindwasser, L.; Budansky, Y.; Leproux, P.; Alfano, R.R. Near-infrared supercontinuum laser beam source in the second and third near-infrared optical windows used to image more deeply through thick tissue as compared with images from a lamp source. *J. Biomed. Opt.* **2015**, *20*, 030501. [CrossRef] [PubMed]
128. Yadav, J.; Rani, A.; Singh, V.; Murari, B.M. Prospects and limitations of non-invasive blood glucose monitoring using near-infrared spectroscopy. *Biomed. Signal. Process. Control* **2015**, *18*, 214–227. [CrossRef]
129. Rostami, E. Glucose and the injured brain-monitored in the neurointensive care unit. *Front. Neurol.* **2014**, *5*. [CrossRef]
130. Pinchefsky, E.F.; Hahn, C.D.; Kamino, D.; Chau, V.; Brant, R.; Moore, A.M.; Tam, E.W.Y. Hyperglycemia and Glucose Variability Are Associated with Worse Brain Function and Seizures in Neonatal Encephalopathy: A Prospective Cohort Study. *J. Pediatr.* **2019**, *209*, 23–32. [CrossRef] [PubMed]
131. Liu, J.; Zhu, C.; Jiang, J.; Xu, K. Scattering-independent glucose absorption measurement using a spectrally resolved reflectance setup with specialized variable source-detector separations. *Biomed. Opt. Express* **2018**, *9*, 5903. [CrossRef]
132. Fuglerud, S.S.; Milenko, K.; Ellingsen, R.; Aksnes, A.; Hjelme, D.R. Feasibility of supercontinuum sources for use in glucose sensing by absorption spectroscopy. In Proceedings of the European Conference on Biomedical Optics 2019, Munich, Germany, 23–25 June 2019; p. 11073_13.
133. Quarto, G.; Farina, A.; Pifferi, A.; Taroni, P.; Miniati, M. Time-resolved optical spectroscopy of the chest: Is it possible to probe the lung? In Proceedings of the European Conference on Biomedical Optics 2013, Munich, Germany, 12–16 May 2013; Taroni, P., Dehghani, H., Eds.; SPIE: Washington, DC, USA, 2013; p. 87990Q.
134. Vignal, C.; Boumans, T.; Montcel, B.; Ramstein, S.; Verhoye, M.; Van Audekerke, J.; Mathevon, N.; Van der Linden, A.; Mottin, S. Measuring brain hemodynamic changes in a songbird: Responses to hypercapnia measured with functional MRI and near-infrared spectroscopy. *Phys. Med. Biol.* **2008**, *53*, 2457–2470. [CrossRef] [PubMed]
135. Wabnitz, H.; Jelzow, A.; Mazurenka, M.; Steinkellner, O.; Macdonald, R.; Pifferi, A.; Torricelli, A.; Contini, D.; Zucchelli, L.M.G.; Spinelli, L.; et al. Performance assessment of time-domain optical brain imagers: A multi-laboratory study. In Proceedings of the SPIE BiOS, San Francisco, CA, USA, 2–7 February 2013; Volume 8583, pp. 85830L–85830L–14.

136. Ferocino, E.; Di Sciacca, G.; Di Sieno, L.; Dalla Mora, A.; Pifferi, A.; Arridge, S.; Martelli, F.; Taroni, P.; Farina, A. Spectral approach to time domain diffuse optical tomography for breast cancer: Validation on meat phantoms. In Proceedings of the European Conference on Biomedical Optics 2019, Munich, Germany, 23–25 June 2019; p. 11074_7.
137. Diop, M.; St. Lawrence, K. Improving the depth sensitivity of time-resolved measurements by extracting the distribution of times-of-flight. *Biomed. Opt. Express* **2013**, *4*, 447. [CrossRef] [PubMed]
138. Nachabé, R.; Evers, D.J.; Hendriks, B.H.W.; Lucassen, G.W.; van der Voort, M.; Rutgers, E.J.; Peeters, M.-J.V.; Van der Hage, J.A.; Oldenburg, H.S.; Wesseling, J.; et al. Diagnosis of breast cancer using diffuse optical spectroscopy from 500 to 1600 nm: Comparison of classification methods. *J. Biomed. Opt.* **2011**, *16*, 087010. [CrossRef]
139. Pifferi, A.; Farina, A.; Torricelli, A.; Quarto, G.; Cubeddu, R.; Taronia, P. Review: Time-domain broadband near infrared spectroscopy of the female breast: A focused review from basic principles to future perspectives. *J. Near Infrared Spectrosc.* **2012**, *20*, 223. [CrossRef]
140. Lindner, C.; Mora, M.; Farzam, P.; Squarcia, M.; Johansson, J.; Weigel, U.M.; Halperin, I.; Hanzu, F.A.; Durduran, T. Diffuse optical characterization of the healthy human thyroid tissue and two pathological case studies. *PLoS ONE* **2016**, *11*, e0147851. [CrossRef]
141. Lange, F.; Tachtsidis, I. Clinical brain monitoring with time domain NIRS: A review and future perspectives. *Appl. Sci.* **2019**, *9*, 1612. [CrossRef]
142. Buttafava, M.; Martinenghi, E.; Tamborini, D.; Contini, D.; Mora, A.D.; Renna, M.; Torricelli, A.; Pifferi, A.; Zappa, F.; Tosi, A. A Compact Two-Wavelength Time-Domain NIRS System Based on SiPM and Pulsed Diode Lasers. *IEEE Photonics J.* **2017**, *9*, 1–14. [CrossRef]
143. Bérubé-Lauzière, Y.; Crotti, M.; Boucher, S.; Ettehadi, S.; Pichette, J.; Rech, I. Prospects on Time-Domain Diffuse Optical Tomography Based on Time-Correlated Single Photon Counting for Small Animal Imaging. *J. Spectrosc.* **2016**, *2016*, 1–23. [CrossRef]
144. Kaynezhad, P.; Mitra, S.; Bale, G.; Bauer, C.; Lingam, I.; Meehan, C.; Avdic-Belltheus, A.; Martinello, K.A.; Bainbridge, A.; Robertson, N.J.; et al. Quantification of the severity of hypoxic-ischemic brain injury in a neonatal preclinical model using measurements of cytochrome-c-oxidase from a miniature broadband-near-infrared spectroscopy system. *Neurophotonics* **2019**, *6*, 1. [CrossRef]
145. Lange, F.; Bale, G.; Kaynezhad, P.; Pollock, R.D.; Stevenson, A.; Tachtsidis, I. Broadband NIRS Cerebral Evaluation of the Hemodynamic and Oxidative State of Cytochrome-c-Oxidase Responses to +Gz Acceleration in Healthy Volunteers. In *Oxygen Transport to Tissue XLI*; Springer: Cham, Switzerland, 2020; Volume 1232.
146. Wu, J.; Zheng, G.; Liu, X.; Qiu, J. Near-infrared laser driven white light continuum generation: Materials, photophysical behaviours and applications. *Chem. Soc. Rev.* **2020**, *49*, 3461–3483. [CrossRef]
147. Alayed, M.; Deen, M. Time-Resolved Diffuse Optical Spectroscopy and Imaging Using Solid-State Detectors: Characteristics, Present Status, and Research Challenges. *Sensors* **2017**, *17*, 2115. [CrossRef]
148. Dalla Mora, A.; Di Sieno, L.; Re, R.; Pifferi, A.; Contini, D. Time-Gated Single-Photon Detection in Time-Domain Diffuse Optics: A Review. *Appl. Sci.* **2020**, *10*, 1101. [CrossRef]
149. Mora, A.D.; Contini, D.; Arridge, S.; Martelli, F.; Tosi, A.; Boso, G.; Farina, A.; Durduran, T.; Martinenghi, E.; Torricelli, A.; et al. Towards next-generation time-domain diffuse optics for extreme depth penetration and sensitivity. *Biomed. Opt. Express* **2015**, *6*, 1749. [CrossRef] [PubMed]
150. Renna, M.; Buttafava, M.; Behera, A.; Zanoletti, M.; Di Sieno, L.; Mora, A.D.; Contini, D.; Tosi, A. Eight-Wavelength, Dual Detection Channel Instrument for Near-Infrared Time-Resolved Diffuse Optical Spectroscopy. *IEEE J. Sel. Top. Quantum Electron.* **2019**, *25*, 1–11. [CrossRef]

Article

Measurement of Adult Human Brain Responses to Breath-Holding by Multi-Distance Hyperspectral Near-Infrared Spectroscopy

Zahida Guerouah [1], Steve Lin [2,3] and Vladislav Toronov [1,2,*]

1. Department of Physics, Faculty of Science, Ryerson University, 350 Victoria Street, Toronto, ON M5B 2K3, Canada; zguerouah@ryerson.ca
2. Institute of Biomedical Engineering, Science and Technology (iBEST), Li Ka-Shing Knowledge Institute, 7th Floor, LKS 735, 209 Victoria Street, Toronto, ON M5B 1T8, Canada; Steve.Lin@unityhealth.to
3. Department of Medicine, University of Toronto, 200 Elizabeth Street, Suite RFE 3-805, Toronto, ON M5G 2C4, Canada
* Correspondence: toronov@ryerson.ca

Abstract: A major limitation of near-infrared spectroscopy (NIRS) is its high sensitivity to the scalp and low sensitivity to the brain of adult humans. In the present work we used multi-distance hyperspectral NIRS (hNIRS) to investigate the optimal source-detector distances, wavelength ranges, and analysis techniques to separate cerebral responses to 30 s breath-holds (BHs) from the responses in the superficial tissue layer in healthy adult humans. We observed significant responses to BHs in the scalp hemodynamics. Cerebral responses to BHs were detected in the cytochrome C oxidase redox (rCCO) at 4 cm without using data from the short-distance channel. Using the data from the 1 cm channel in the two-layer regression algorithm showed that cerebral hemodynamic and rCCO responses also occurred at 3 cm. We found that the waveband 700–900 nm was optimal for the detection of cerebral responses to BHs in adults.

Keywords: near-infrared spectroscopy; brain; BOLD signal; breath-holding; cytochrome C oxidase

1. Introduction

Near-infrared spectroscopy (NIRS) was proposed for human brain measurements in 1970s [1]. It has also been considered for clinical monitoring of cerebral status during various medical conditions in adults, such as cardiac surgeries, cardiac arrest, and traumatic brain injury [2]. However, in such conditions significant circulatory and metabolic changes occur in the entire body, including the scalp, where NIRS sensitivity is maximal [3,4]. In general, high sensitivity to the scalp and low sensitivity to the brain of adult humans remains a main problem of NIRS in spite of numerous attempts to resolve it using continuous-wave [5], time-domain [6], and frequency-domain approaches [7]. In particular, in several papers the combination of long and short source-detector channels was proposed and investigated [5,8–12]. Other aspects of cerebral NIRS requiring investigation include optimization of the spectrum of wavelengths [13–15], and of the range of source-detector distances [14–16] for specific categories of subjects and patients—children, adults, and seniors. In the present work we approached the above aspects of cerebral NIRS using multi-distance hyperspectral NIRS (hNIRS).

Apart from the ability to measure the optical properties of tissue at all NIR wavelengths simultaneously, hNIRS is the most robust technique to spectrally separate hemoglobin and redox cytochrome C oxidase (rCCO) changes [4,17,18]. An increase in rCCO signal corresponds to an increase in oxidized CCO and an equal decrease in reduced CCO. While rCCO is a direct marker of cellular oxygen metabolism, the robust measurement of rCCO is much more challenging than measurement of the blood parameters due to the much lower concentration of CCO than of hemoglobin. Therefore, the development and validation of the methodology for rCCO measurements remains a hot topic of NIRS research. Reference [18] provide comprehensive reviews of the physiological significance, and of the history and various aspects of measurements of cerebral rCCO. A review of multiple possible factors that can change rCCO in the brain (changes in oxygen tension, ATP, NADH, etc.) is available in [19].

In this work we used hNIRS to study the possibility to measure specific cerebral autoregulation changes concomitant with systemic changes at source-detector distances of 1 cm, 3 cm, and 4 cm in healthy adults during breath-holding (BH) respiratory challenges. Since BH was proposed as a clinical paradigm to assess cerebral status in various clinical conditions such as stroke, concussion, etc. [20–22], the dynamics of cerebral responses to BH have been studied both by NIRS [23,24] and functional magnetic resonance imaging (fMRI) [25,26], which allows for a direct comparison of our results with other studies.

2. Materials and Methods

The study was conducted according to the guidelines of the Declaration of Helsinki, and approved by the Research Ethics Board of Ryerson University (REB: 2008-003-1, 4 May 2015).

2.1. Measurement Setup

An hNIRS custom sensor was placed on the left forehead over the Fp1 position according to the International 10–20 system [27] for the entire measurement procedure (see Figure 1). The distance between two sources was 8 mm (Figure 1b). According to the Monte-Carlo simulation of the light propagation in the adult human head [3] and to the fMRI studies [25,26], with such a geometry the light from both sources collected at 3 cm and 4 cm interrogated the cortical region which was expected to show the same dynamics during BH.

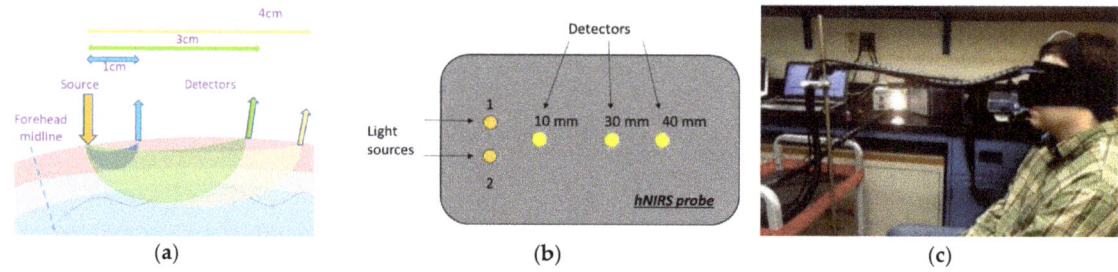

Figure 1. hNIRS measurement setup: (**a**) approximate interrogated volumes in the scalp, skull, and brain; (**b**) optical sensor layout; and (**c**) subject position.

The spectra were collected at the sampling rate of 2 Hz by three fiber optic spectrometers—AvaSpec (Avantes, CO, USA) and QE 65000 and USB 4000 (Ocean Optics, Dunedin, FL, USA) at 4, 3, and 1 cm, respectively, to separate the extracerebral and cerebral measurements. The spectrometers were tested on the same phantom and on a human forearm muscle to ensure that at the same distance they measured the same absorbance within the 700–1000 nm wavelength range. AvaSoft-Full software (Avantes, CO, USA) was used to collect data from the AvaSpec spectrometer (4 cm), and The Spectra Suite (Ocean Optics, FL, USA) software was used to collect the broadband continuous-wave hNIRS data from both Ocean Optics spectrometers with dark-signal correction. Data acquired at 1 cm represented the extra-cerebral layer (mostly scalp). Data acquired at 3 cm and 4 cm channels represented a combined extracerebral and cerebral tissue volume. The common spectral range of these spectrometers was from 650 to 1024 nm. The spectrometers at 4 cm and 3 cm had a high signal-to-noise ratio (over 1000:1 single acquisition) and the slit width of 0.5 mm to provide the sensitivity required to measure light at large distance from the source. Three custom-made 2-m-long optical fiber bundles (each made of seven 0.5 NA, 400 µm core-diameter multimode polymer-clad fibers with broad UV/VIS/NIR spectral range of 400 to 2200 nm Thorlabs, NJ, USA) connected spectrometers with the patient's head. Two other optical fiber bundles were used to connect the probe with a halogen lamp light source (Fiber-Lite Dc 950H Fiber Optic Illuminator, Dolan-Jenner, MA, USA). The source light was injected into the tissue at two symmetric scalp locations (Figure 1b) in order to increase the total light power without exceeding the maximum permissible exposure.

2.2. Breath-Holding Paradigm

Data were obtained from 12 healthy adult participants (seven males, five females, 25–55 years old). All participants gave informed consent before participation and the experiment was performed according to Ryerson University Research Ethics protocol. Participants were audibly cued to perform a 30 s BH at the end of expiration. BH was repeated three times (60–90 s, 180–210 s, and 300–330 s from the beginning of the recording) with 90 s rest intervals. Long time intervals between BHs were used to avoid resonance induction of systemic Mayer waves in arterial blood pressure [28,29]. All data sets including the baseline periods before and after BHs were acquired during 10 min.

2.3. Data Processing

All our custom signal processing methods were implemented in MATLAB (Mathworks, Natick, MA, USA, Version R2020b). At the pre-processing stage the data from all spectrometers were resampled in both time and spectral domains to the time step of 0.5 s and wavelength step of 1 nm between 650 and 1024 nm, filtered in the time domain using a band-pass filter with the window of 0.01–0.3 Hz, and smoothed in the spectral domain with the median filter of the 20 nm width. To analyze the chromophores, we used two custom data processing approaches. Our first algorithm was based on the analytical solution to the diffusion equation [30,31] for the semi-infinite homogeneous medium. This allows for measuring the bulk absolute concentrations of tissue HbO$_2$ and HHb, and changes in rCCO concentration without accounting for the layered tissue structure. The baseline concentrations of HbO$_2$ and HHb were calculated by performing a non-linear least square fitting [30,31] of the measured absorbance spectrum at each moment of time by the analytical solution to the diffusion equation, in which the optical absorption coefficient $\mu_a(\lambda)$ was modeled as

$$\mu_a(\lambda) = [\text{Hb}]\varepsilon(\lambda)_{\text{Hb}} + [\text{HbO}_2]\varepsilon(\lambda)_{\text{HbO}_2} + \eta(\lambda) \tag{1}$$

According to Beer–Lambert law, the reduced scattering coefficient $\mu_s'(\lambda)$ as a function of wavelength λ was modeled using the power law as described in [30]. In Equation (1) and below the square brackets denote concentrations measured in micromoles (µM), $\eta(\lambda)$ is the absorption by water assuming 80% water concentration. The temporal changes in the hemoglobin concentrations HbO$_2$, Hb, and rCOO were resolved using a two-step data-fitting algorithm [30,31] (also based on the same analytical solution to the diffusion equation) by relating changes in HbO$_2$, Hb, and rCOO to the changes in the optical absorbance as

$$\Delta\mu_a(\lambda,t) = \Delta[\text{Hb}](t)\varepsilon(\lambda)_{\text{Hb}} + \Delta[\text{HbO}_2](t)\varepsilon(\lambda)_{\text{HbO}_2} + \Delta[\text{CCO}](t)\varepsilon(\lambda)_{\text{cco}}, \tag{2}$$

where $\varepsilon(\lambda)_x$ were the spectra of the extinction coefficients of HbO$_2$, Hb, and rCCO (see Figure 2) [30,31].

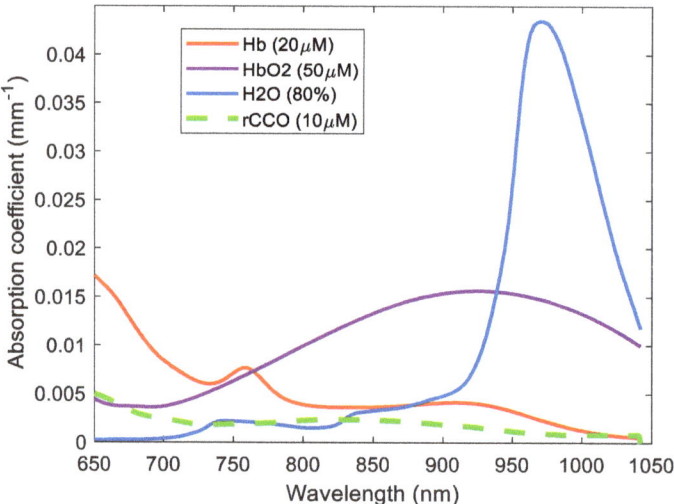

Figure 2. Absorption spectra of HHb, HbO$_2$, H2O, and rCCO.

The data-fitting was performed in two steps: first Δ[HbO$_2$] and Δ[HHb] were calculated assuming Δ[CCO] = 0, and after that Δ[CCO] was calculated and retained non-zero only if the addition of Δ[CCO] resulted in an improvement in the fit quality of at least 20% in terms of the norm of residuals. Such a stepwise regression worked as an adaptive filter reducing the noise in the time-course of rCCO without suppressing changes recognized from significant spectral distortions corresponding to $\varepsilon(\lambda)_{cco}$. Additional details on recovering the absolute values and changes of chromophore concentrations from the hNIRS data can be found in [32,33].

As the fraction of oxygenated hemoglobin relative to the total hemoglobin in the blood, the cerebral tissue saturation of oxygen was calculated as:

$$tSO_2 = \frac{[HbO_2]}{[HbO_2] + [Hb]}(\%). \quad (3)$$

In order to assess differences between the cerebral and scalp responses to BH we used another common NIRS model—the modified Lambert–Beer law for a two-layer medium [32,33]. This model assumes that at any moment of time, t, the absorbance measured at 1 cm and at the wavelength λ can be related to the changes of the absorption coefficient of the scalp only $\Delta\mu_{a,s}(\lambda, t)$:

$$\Delta OD_{1cm}(\lambda, t) = L_{s\ 1cm}\Delta\mu_{a,s}(\lambda, t), \quad (4)$$

where $L_{s\ 1cm}$ is the optical pathlength in the scalp at 1 cm, and the absorbance at 3 cm and 4 cm could be expressed as

$$\Delta OD_{3cm}(\lambda, t) = L_{s\ 3cm}\Delta\mu_{a,s}(\lambda, t) + L_{c\ 3cm}\Delta\mu_{a,c}(\lambda, t) \quad (5)$$

$$\Delta OD_{4cm}(\lambda, t) = L_{s\ 4cm}\Delta\mu_{a,s}(\lambda, t) + L_{c\ 4cm}\Delta\mu_{a,c}(\lambda, t) \quad (6)$$

where $\Delta\mu_{a,c}(\lambda, t)$ is the change in the cerebral absorption coefficient, $L_{s\ 3cm}$ and $L_{s\ 4cm}$ are the scalp partial pathlength at 3 cm and 4 cm, respectively, and $L_{c\ 3cm}$ and $L_{c\ 4cm}$ are the cerebral partial pathlength at 3 cm and 4 cm, respectively. Since the pathlengths in Equations (4)–(6) were specific for every individual and unknown, $\Delta\mu_{a,s}$ could not be algebraically excluded to find $\Delta\mu_{a,c}$. However, since Equations (4) and (5) were linear with respect to the common time-dependent $\Delta\mu_{a,s}(\lambda, t)$ and $\Delta\mu_{a,c}(\lambda, t)$, for every wavelength,

λ, one could exclude the time-course common with $\Delta\mu_{a,s}(\lambda,t)$ from $\Delta OD_{3cm}(\lambda,t)$ and $\Delta OD_{4cm}(\lambda,t)$. Indeed, one could rewrite Equations (5) and (6) in the form

$$\Delta OD_{3cm}(\lambda,t) = L_{c\,3cm}\delta\mu_{a,c}(\lambda,t) + (L_{c\,3cm} + L_{s\,3cm})\left(L_{(s\,1cm)}\right)^{-1}\Delta OD_{1cm}(\lambda,t) \quad (7)$$

$$\Delta OD_{4cm}(\lambda,t) = L_{c\,4cm}\delta\mu_{a,c}(\lambda,t) + (L_{c\,4cm} + L_{s\,4cm})\left(L_{(s\,1cm)}\right)^{-1}\Delta OD_{1cm}(\lambda,t) \quad (8)$$

where

$$\delta\mu_{a,c}(\lambda,t) = \Delta\mu_{a,c}(\lambda,t) - \Delta\mu_{a,s}(\lambda,t) \quad (9)$$

represents the difference between the cerebral and scalp responses to BH. Note that Equations (7) and (8) are linear with respect to $\Delta OD_{1cm}(\lambda,t)$ and $\delta\mu_{a,c}(\lambda,t)$, and also we expect that the latter functions of time and wavelength will be uncorrelated in the time domain. Therefore the time-domain linear regression coefficients between $\Delta OD_{1cm}(\lambda,t)$ and $\Delta OD_{3cm}(\lambda,t)$ and between $\Delta OD_{1cm}(\lambda,t)$ and $\Delta OD_{4cm}(\lambda,t)$ should be close to $\beta_{1,3\,cm} \approx (L_{c\,3cm} + L_{s\,3cm})\left(L_{(s\,1cm)}\right)^{-1}$ and $\beta_{1,4\,cm} \approx (L_{c\,4cm} + L_{s\,4cm})\left(L_{(s\,1cm)}\right)^{-1}$, respectively. Then, by subtracting $\beta_{1,3\,cm}(\lambda)\Delta OD_{1cm}(\lambda,t)$ and $\beta_{1,4\,cm}(\lambda)\Delta OD_{1cm}(\lambda,t)$ from Equations (7) and (8) we obtain:

$$\delta OD_{3cm}(\lambda,t) \approx L_{c\,3cm}\delta\mu_{a,c}(\lambda,t), \text{ and } \delta OD_{4cm}(\lambda,t) \approx L_{c\,4cm}\delta\mu_{a,c}(\lambda,t) \quad (10)$$

Note that at all wavelengths the true cerebral response to BH could have a component close to the scalp response. Therefore, $\delta OD_{3,4\,cm}(\lambda,t)$ represent not the pure time-course of the cerebral absorption coefficient, but rather the difference between the cerebral and scalp absorption time-courses.

In accordance with Equation (2) one could model $\delta OD_{3,4\,cm}(\lambda,t)$ as a linear combination of the contributions from $\delta[\text{Hb}](t)$, $\delta[\text{HbO}_2](t)$, and $\delta[\text{rCCO}](t)$:

$$\delta OD_{3,4\,cm}(\lambda,t) \sim \delta[\text{Hb}](t)\varepsilon(\lambda)_{\text{Hb}} + \delta[\text{HbO}_2](t)\varepsilon(\lambda)_{\text{HbO}_2} + \delta[\text{rCCO}](t)\varepsilon(\lambda)_{\text{rcco}}. \quad (11)$$

By applying the stepwise linear regression spectral unmixing to the linear model (Equation (9)) (where the regressors are the extinction coefficients $\varepsilon(\lambda)_x$) one could obtain the specific cerebral changes $\delta[\text{Hb}](t)$, $\delta[\text{HbO}_2](t)$, and $\delta[\text{rCCO}](t)$, whose time-courses represent the differences between the cerebral and scalp responses in HHb, HbO_2, and rCCO, respectively. In this spectral unmixing step the initial regression model did not include $\delta[\text{rCCO}](t)$. It was added to the model at the second step of the stepwise regression only if the p-value corresponding to non-zero $\delta[\text{rCCO}](t)$ was greater than 0.05.

In addition, we also used Equation (10) to calculate the specific cerebral response in the total hemoglobin $\delta[t\text{Hb}]$. However, $\delta[t\text{Hb}]$ was calculated not by using the spectral unmixing, but by directly using Equation (10) around 800 nm since at this wavelength $\varepsilon_{\text{Hb}} = \varepsilon_{\text{HbO}_2}$. Since near 800 nm $\varepsilon(\lambda)_{rcco}$ is greater than ε_{Hb}, $\delta[t\text{Hb}]$ could include a crosstalk with $\delta[\text{rCCO}](t)$.

Since the values of cerebral pathlengths $L_{c\,3cm}$ and $L_{c\,4cm}$ were unknown, for the quantitative comparison in µM with the responses obtained using the homogeneous tissue model (explained above) we normalized $\delta[\text{Hb}](t)$, $\delta[\text{HbO}_2](t)$, and $\delta[\text{rCCO}](t)$ to the pathlength corresponding to the homogeneous tissue equal to the product of the differential pathlength factor (known be close to 6 for the mid-age human forehead [34]) and the source-detector distance.

2.4. Statistical Analysis

In the individual subject data the peak magnitudes of responses in $\Delta[\text{Hb}]$, $\Delta[\text{HbO}_2]$, and $\Delta[\text{CCO}]$, and in $\delta[\text{Hb}]$, $\delta[\text{HbO}_2]$, and $\delta[\text{CCO}]$ were measured as the difference between the time average over ± 5 s around each peak time (see Table 1) and the average over 20 s just before BHs. These samples were checked for normality (positively) and further tested by the one-sample *t*-test (*ttest* MATLAB function) and *p*-values reported in Tables 1 and 2. In addition, the differences in response magnitudes among three BH episodes were analyzed using *ranova* MATLAB function (repeated measures analysis of variance, RM ANOVA).

Table 1. Cross-subject average peak magnitudes, *p*-values, and peak times obtained from the homogeneous semi-infinite diffusion analysis. The peak magnitudes were measured from the 20 s averaged values before BHs. The peak times measured from the beginning of BHs were found in the averaged traces shown in Figure 4 with the errors estimated as the mean absolute deviation from the individual data.

		HbO$_2$: Peak, *p*-Value, and Peak Times			
		1st BH	2nd BH	3rd BH	Cumulative
1 cm	Δ(μM)	5.7 $\pm$ 1.4, 0.01	6.3 $\pm$ 1.5, 0.02	3.7 $\pm$ 0.9, 0.001	5.2 $\pm$ 0.8, 0.000002
	t(s)	25.4 $\pm$ 3.5	28.6 $\pm$ 3.7	30.5 $\pm$ 4.3	28.2 $\pm$ 2.3
3 cm	Δ(μM)	2.8 $\pm$ 0.6, 0.04	2.9 $\pm$ 0.6, 0.01	2.1 $\pm$ 0.5, 0.01	2.6 $\pm$ 0.3, 0.000002
	t(s)	33.6 $\pm$ 3.6	29.6 $\pm$ 2.8	31.6 $\pm$ 3.3	31.6 $\pm$ 1.9
4 cm	Δ(μM)	0.2 $\pm$ 0.06	0.2 $\pm$ 0.1, 0.01	0.2 $\pm$ 0.1, 0.3	0.2 $\pm$ 0.07, 0.001
	t(s)	28.0 $\pm$ 5.4	28.8 $\pm$ 4.1	26.6 $\pm$ 4.3	27.9 $\pm$ 1.3
		rCCO: Peak, *p*-Value, and Peak Times			
		1st BH	2nd BH	3rd BH	Cumulative
4 cm	Δ*10^{-2}	1.1 $\pm$ 0.2, 0.01	0.9 $\pm$ 0.1, 0.05	0.8 $\pm$ 0.2, 0.04	0.9 $\pm$ 0.1, 0.00007
	t(s)	24.4 $\pm$ 3.9	29.4 $\pm$ 5.4	27.6 $\pm$ 4.7	27.1 $\pm$ 2.5
		HHb: Peak, *p*-Value, and Peak Times			
		1st BH	2nd BH	3rd BH	Cumulative
1 cm	Δ(μM)	1.9 $\pm$ 0.4, 0.017	2.1 $\pm$ 0.4, 0.015	1.9 $\pm$ 0.3, 0.002	2.0 $\pm$ 0.2, 0.00001
	t(s)	35.0 $\pm$ 3.8	36.5 $\pm$ 4.1	42.5 $\pm$ 3.8	38.5 $\pm$ 4.0
3 cm	Δ(μM)	0.7 $\pm$ 0.3, 0.02	0.6 $\pm$ 0.2, 0.01	0.6 $\pm$ 0.2, 0.04	0.6 $\pm$ 0.06, 0.0003
	t(s)	33.0 $\pm$ 4.3	32.5 $\pm$ 4.6	34.5 $\pm$ 5.1	33.3 $\pm$ 1.3
4 cm	Δ(μM)	0.4 $\pm$ 0.1, 0.02	0.3 $\pm$ 0.1, 0.6	0.4 $\pm$ 0.1, 0.04	0.4 $\pm$ 0.06, 0.008
	t(s)	32.2 $\pm$ 5.7	31.7 $\pm$ 6.3	34.3 $\pm$ 4.9	32.7 $\pm$ 3.3

Table 2. Cross-subject average peak magnitudes and *p*-values obtained from the two-layer regression analysis. The peak magnitudes were measured from the 20 s averaged values before BHs.

		HbO$_2$: Peak, *p*-Value			
		1st BH	2nd BH	3rd BH	Cumulative
		Peak, *p*-Value	Peak, *p*-Value	Peak, *p*-Value	
3 cm	Δ(μM)	0.2 $\pm$ 0.3, 0.05	0.1 $\pm$ 0.3, 0.2	0.2 $\pm$ 0.3, 0.2	0.2 $\pm$ 0.3, 0.007
4 cm	Δ(μM)	$-$0.07 $\pm$ 0.09, 0.2	$-$0.03 $\pm$ 0.1, 0.3	$-$0.02 $\pm$ 0.09, 0.4	$-$0.04 $\pm$ 0.1, 0.01
		rCCO: Peak, *p*-Value			
		1st BH	2nd BH	3rd BH	Cumulative
3 cm	Δ(μM)	0.6 $\pm$ 0.6, 0.005	0.6 $\pm$ 0.7, 0.03	0.7 $\pm$ 0.5, 0.002	0.6 $\pm$ 0.6, 0.000002
4 cm	Δ(μM)	0.2 $\pm$ 0.3, 0.03	0.1 $\pm$ 0.2, 0.03	0.2 $\pm$ 0.2, 0.001	0.2 $\pm$ 0.6, 0.000009
		HHb: Peak, *p*-Value			
		1st BH	2nd BH	3rd BH	Cumulative
3 cm	Δ(μM)	0.3 $\pm$ 0.4, 0.06	0.2 $\pm$ 0.4, 0.1	0.1 $\pm$ 0.5, 0.4	0.2 $\pm$ 0.4, 0.01
4 cm	Δ(μM)	0.1 $\pm$ 0.1, 0.006	0.05 $\pm$ 0.09, 0.1	0.05 $\pm$ 0.1, 0.13	0.08 $\pm$ 0.1, 0.0004
		tHB: Peak, *p*-Value			
		1st BH	2nd BH	3rd BH	Cumulative
3 cm	Δ(μM)	1.4 $\pm$ 1.7, 0.02	1.4 $\pm$ 1.4, 0.005	1.4 $\pm$ 1.7, 0.01	1.4 $\pm$ 1.6, 0.000005
4 cm	Δ(μM)	0.4 $\pm$ 0.5, 0.02	0.3 $\pm$ 0.4, 0.03	0.4 $\pm$ 0.5, 0.02	0.4 $\pm$ 0.4, 0.00003

3. Results

Figure 3 shows the assessment of de-noised signals in all three channels and at all wavelengths in terms of the cross-subject averaged temporal correlation (first and second rows), temporal logarithmic signal means (third row, used for the data quality assessment), and temporal standard deviations (fourth row).

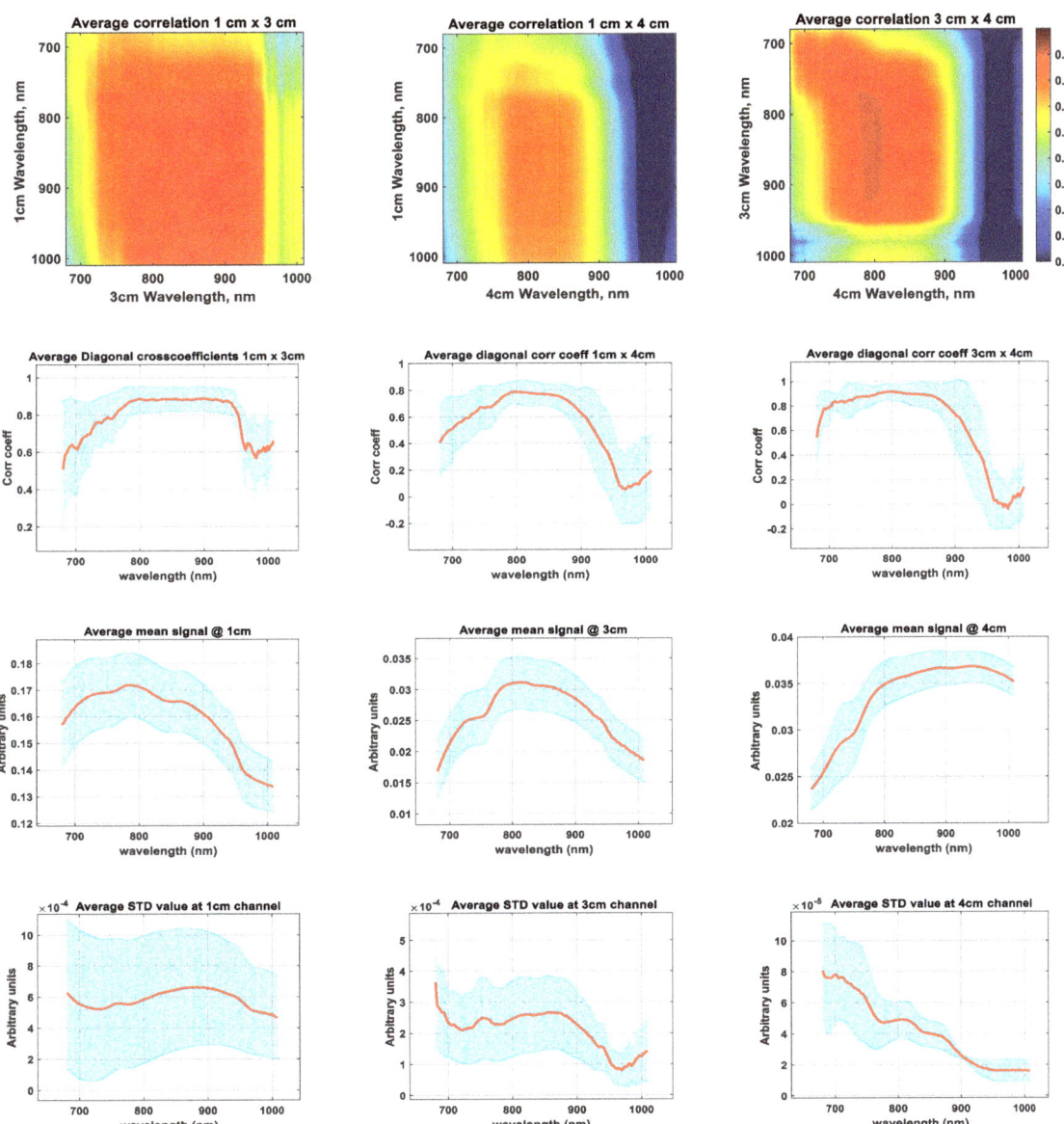

Figure 3. Hyperspectral signal analysis: cross-subject averaged correlation, temporal means, and temporal standard deviations for signals from 1 cm, 3 cm, and 4 cm channels. Blue color shows the cross-subject standard deviations.

Since the noise was filtered out, the latter represent the average magnitude of changes at different wavelengths. The correlation coefficient maps (first row) show that signals at all wavelengths from 700 nm to over 900 nm and in all channels were positively correlated. The latter means that there were no pairs of signals at any wavelengths from 700 nm to 900 nm and in any channels where temporal changes occurred simultaneously in opposite directions. Also from the correlation maps and same-wavelength correlation plots (second row) one could see that all signals between 750 nm and 900 nm were highly correlated (correlation coefficient > 0.6). This high correlation occurred because, as shown in [3], at both 3 and 4 cm the optical pathlength in the extracerebral tissue was several times longer than in the brain, and therefore the scalp contribution was high at both 4 and 3 cm channels. Correlations were low for the wavelengths longer than 900 nm in the 4 cm channel. While the mean signal value in the 4 cm channel at these wavelengths was high (third row), the amplitude of changes (fourth row) was small. This lack of changes should be due to fact that at longer wavelengths the partial optical pathlengths in the tissues where the changes occurred (scalp and brain) was shorter than at wavelengths below 900 nm, and at the 4 cm source-detector separation the light of wavelengths greater than 900 nm mostly interrogated the volume which belongs to the skull where no changes occurred. For the above reasons the further analysis was performed using the waveband from 750 nm to 900 nm.

Figure 4 shows the cross-subject averaged changes in [HbO_2], [HHb], [rCCO], and [rSO_2] measured at 1 cm, 3 cm, and 4 cm using the homogeneous tissue model and 750–900 nm waveband. One could see that the hemoglobin signals showed responses to BHs in all channels, while rCCO exhibited clear responses only at 4 cm. Table 1 presents the average amplitude, p-values, and temporal values characteristic for the chromophore responses to BHs. In addition to Figures 4 and 5 provides a direct comparison of the hemoglobin time-courses at 1 cm and 4 cm and shows a return to the baseline 4 min after BHs.

As shown in Figures 4 and 5, and also from the peak times for HbO_2 in Table 1 the time-courses of HbO_2 responses appeared similar in all channels. The common features of HHb responses to BHs in 1 cm and 3 cm channels were the initial dips followed by quick increases peaking up 4–10 s after the end of BH. The depth of initial dips was much greater in the 1 cm channel than in 3 cm and 4 cm channels (Figure 5b). However, the magnitudes of these dips measured from the HHb levels just before BH were statistically insignificant ($p > 0.05$). The HHb peak times were longest for the 1 cm channel (about 9 s after the end of BH, see Table 1). Much earlier peaks and faster falls in the HHb responses at 4 cm compared to those features at 1 cm (Figure 5b, Table 1) might indicate a prevalence of the cerebral component in the 4 cm HHb responses. In particular, the faster falls of HHb at 4 cm than at 1 cm could be due to the cerebral autoregulation restoring the oxygen concentration in the brain faster than in extracerebral tissues. In Figure 4 one can also see that at 3 cm the HHb responses were intermediate between those measured at 1 cm and 4 cm.

The rCCO signals from the 1 cm and 3 cm channels showed no clear responses to BHs. In contrast, at 4 cm the rCCO responses were very clear (Figures 4 and 5c), which also might indicate that these responses belonged solely to the cerebral tissue. Each rCCO fall after the end of BH was quickly followed by a rebound which also could be a result of the faster restoration of the oxygen supply in the brain than in other tissues. Note that rCCO peak changes had about 10 times smaller magnitudes than HbO_2 and HHb changes (Table 1), which was in agreement with the fact that the concentration of CCO in the brain is approximately 10 times smaller than the concentration of hemoglobin.

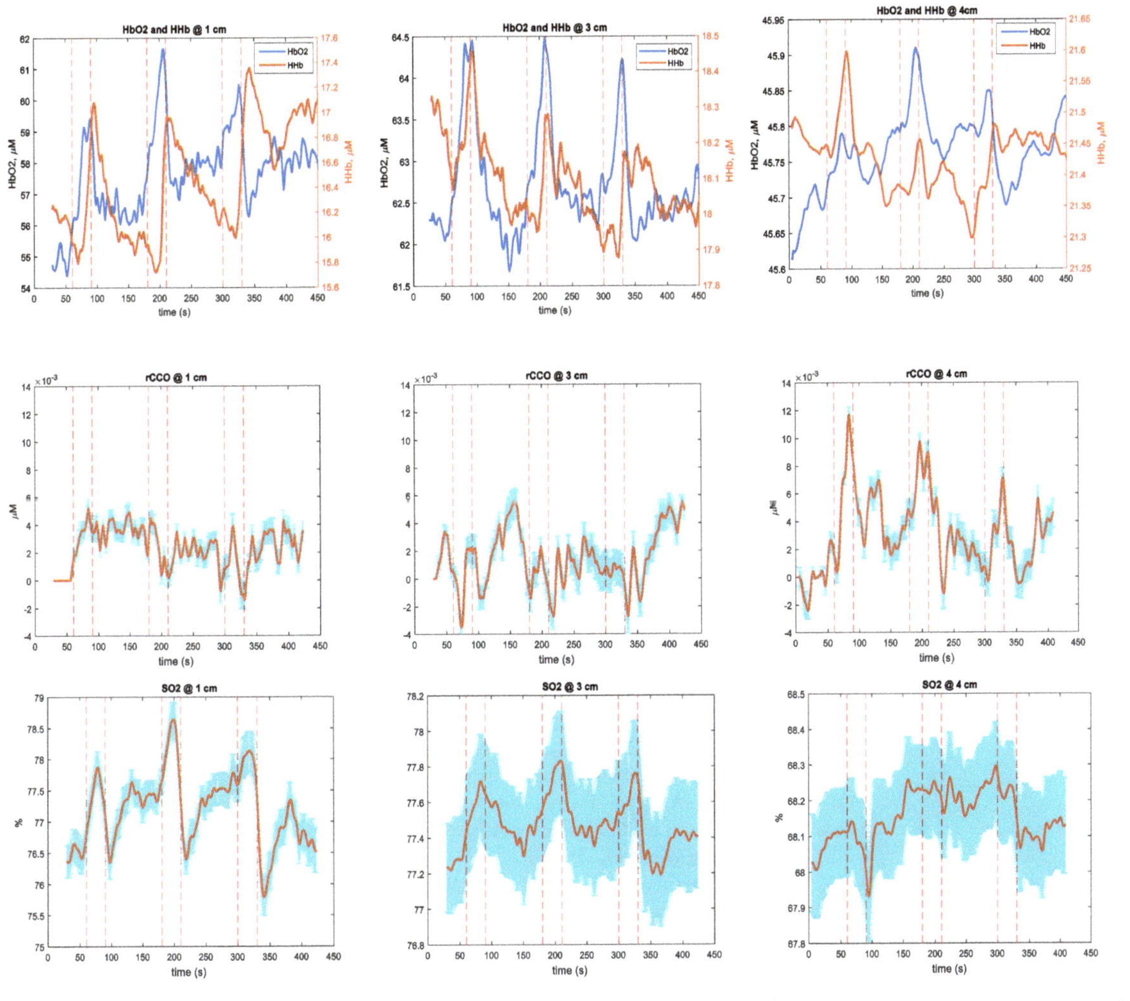

Figure 4. Cross-subject averaged changes in [HbO2], [HHb], and [rCCO], and regional SO_2 measured at 1 cm, 3 cm, and 4 cm using the homogeneous tissue model and 750–900nm waveband. Blue color shows the cross-subject standard deviations.

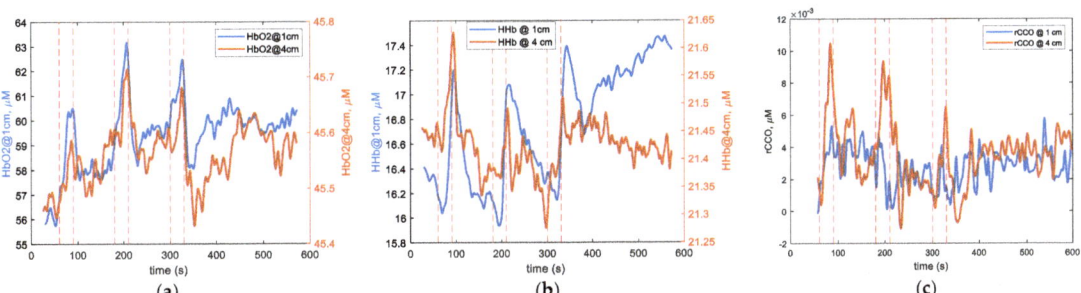

Figure 5. Cross-subject averaged temporal traces of [HbO_2] (**a**), [HHb] (**b**), and [rCCO] (**c**) showing a comparison of 1 cm and 4 cm time-courses and a return to the baseline 4 min after BHs.

In Figure 4 the SO_2 time-course at 4 cm was also very different from those at 1 cm and 3 cm, which were very similar to each other by showing SO_2 increases characteristic for the scalp tissue. However, the quick SO_2 falls at 4 cm at the end of each BH should not be interpreted as the failure of cerebral autoregulation but rather, these falls resulted from the smaller magnitude of the HbO_2 increase than of the HHb increase due to the difference in the partial volume of the skull interrogated by light at shorter and longer wavelengths. From Table 1 one can see that the magnitudes of HbO_2 and HHb responses to BHs decreased with the distance. The reason for this was the application of the homogeneous model to the measurements of the inhomogeneous tissue, which included bone, where almost no blood was present. With the increase of the distance the partial volume of the bone increased leading to the underestimation of the magnitudes of HbO_2 and HHb responses to BHs at 3 cm and 4 cm.

The cumulative p-values in Table 1 show that all included responses were statistically significant at $p < 0.05$ when the results of all three BHs were combined. HbO_2 and HHb responses to each individual BH were significant at 1 cm and at 3 cm. Unlike HbO_2 and HHb, at 4 cm, rCCO responses to each individual BH were statistically significant. Although the average peak values for different BHs in Table 1 were different, RM ANOVA analysis did not show statistical significance of these differences.

As explained above, in order to reveal differences between responses to BHs measured in different channels we performed time-spectral linear regression analysis. For the regression analysis the range of wavelengths was limited to 750–900 nm where the highest correlation between different channels was detected (see Figure 3). Figure 6 shows the cross-subject average correlation and standard deviations spectra of signals from the 3 cm and 4 cm channels after regressing out changes measured at the 1 cm channel. One could see that the correlation coefficient for all wavelengths in both channels was greater than 0.6 between 750 nm and 900 nm. The correlation coefficient for the same wavelengths in both channels (corresponding to the diagonal of the correlation map in Figure 6) was particularly high for all wavelengths. This high correlation indicated that after regressing out the superficial changes, both 3 cm and 4 cm channels exhibited very similar time-courses at all wavelengths. Also in Figure 6 one can see that the spectra of average amplitudes of changes (measured by SDs) were similar in shape to those before regression (shown in Figure 3). They showed peaks at the HHb and rCCO absorption maxima around 760 nm and 830 nm, respectively, (compare with Figure 2), and decreased at wavelengths longer than 870 nm, corresponding to maximum HbO_2 absorption. Therefore, after the regression the HbO_2 changes should have smaller magnitudes than the HHb and rCCO responses.

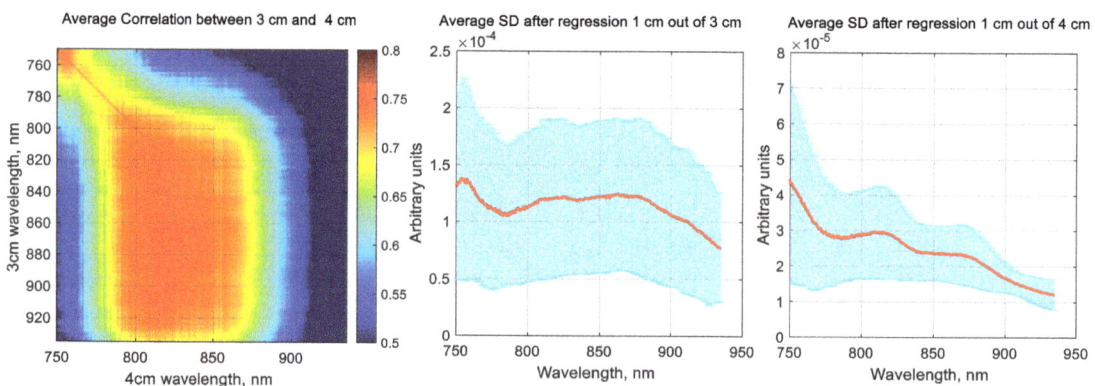

Figure 6. Cross-subject average correlation and standard deviation spectra of signals from the 3 cm and 4 cm channels after regressing out changes measured at the 1 cm channel.

In Figure 7 the green and blue curves show the cross-subject averaged changes in HbO_2, HHb, tHB, and rCCO calculated by applying the spectral-domain regression to the residuals after regressing out the in time-domain the changes measured at the 1 cm channel from the signals measured at the 3 cm and 4 cm channels, respectively. The tHB changes were computed by averaging changes in the 5 nm waveband around 800 nm where the HHb- and HbO_2-specific absorptions were equal. Note that the changes in Figure 7 show the differences in the time-courses of changes in the deep and superficial tissues. (Note that signals measured at different channels never changed in opposite directions, which follows from the correlation analysis shown in Figure 3 and explained above.) In particular, the rising slopes seen on the curves in Figure 7 correspond to the time intervals when changes measured at 3 or 4 cm increased faster than changes measured at 1 cm. Conversely, the curves in Figure 6 show negative slopes during the times when changes measured at long-distance channels decreased faster than changes measured at the 1 cm channel. The fact that the HbO_2 responses to BHs were not very clear means that the time-courses of $[HbO_2]$ changes in the superficial and cerebral tissues were similar. (The "noise" seen in Figure 7 was mostly due to the respiratory sinus arrhythmia between BHs). In Figure 7 one can also see that the peak times of [HHb], [tHB], and [rCCO] responses during all three BH episodes were between 15 and 25 s after the BH onsets, which was similar to the peak times of rCCO responses shown in Figure 4, but very different from the peak times of HbO_2 and HHb responses shown in Figure 4, which never occurred earlier than 26 s from the beginning of a BH episode (see also Table 1). Some details of the HHb, tHB, and rCCO responses in Figure 7 were quite different. In particular, during BH episodes, the HHb curves showed initial dips during the first 10–15 s turning into the fast increases after that. During the same initial periods of BHs the tHB curves showed steady positive changes, while rCCO curves showed almost no changes during the first 10 s. These differences indicated that the responses to BHs in Figure 7 indeed corresponded to different chromophores and did not result from a crosstalk between different NIR wavelengths. The fact that in Figure 7 the curves corresponding to the 4 cm channel showed similar changes to the curves corresponding to the 3 cm channel but with much smaller magnitudes was due to the overall smaller magnitudes of changes at 4 cm as shown in Figure 3 and explained above.

In addition, the red curves in Figure 7 correspond to regressing out the 3 cm changes from the 4 cm changes. The fact that these curves show almost no changes means that after regressing out the changes due to the contribution from the superficial tissues, the time-courses of changes at all wavelengths in both 3 cm and 4 cm channels were very similar, which was also in agreement with the high correlation between signals from these channels at all wavelengths as shown in Figure 6.

Table 2 shows that HHb-, tHb-, and rCCO-specific cerebral responses to each individual BH were significant at both 3 cm and at 4 cm. rCCO responses showed highest significance ($p < 0.03$) among all chromophores. HbO_2-specific cerebral responses to individual BHs were not significant at 3 cm or at 4 cm. RM ANOVA analysis did not reveal statistical significance of differences in responses to different BH trials.

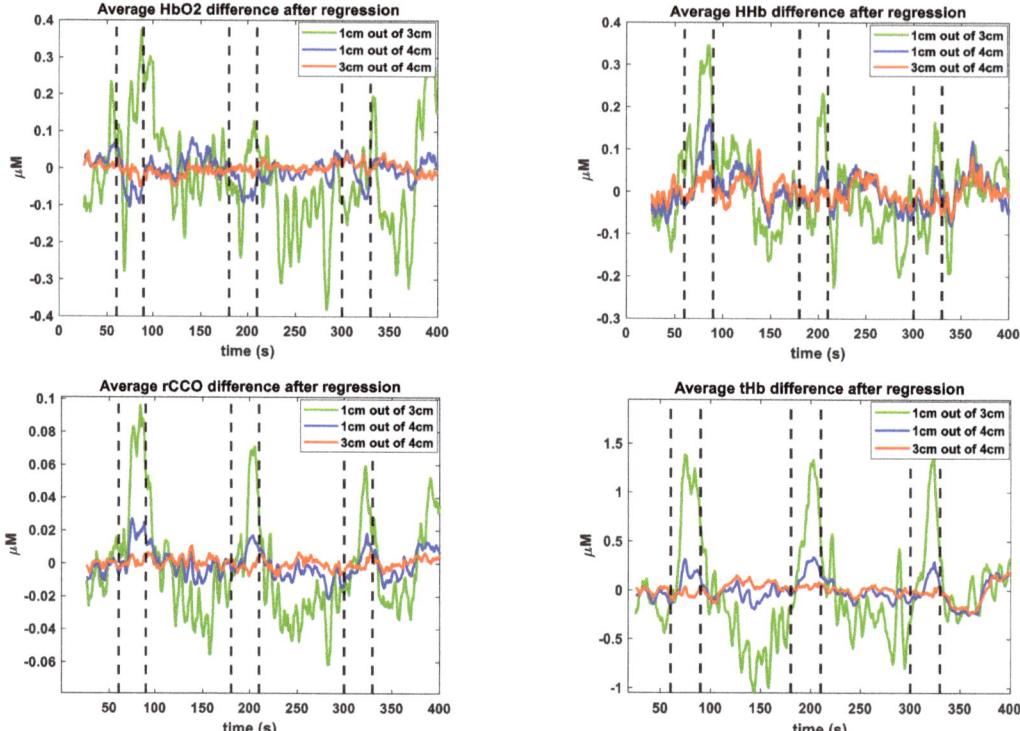

Figure 7. Cross-subject averaged changes in [HbO$_2$], [HHb], [tHB], and [rCCO] calculated from the time-domain regression residuals using stepwise linear regression in spectral domain.

4. Discussion

Our results showed that BHs induced significant hemodynamic responses in all three channels including the 1 cm channel, which mainly interrogated the scalp and partially the skull. Hemodynamic responses measured by the 3 cm channel were quite similar to those measured at 1 cm. In Figures 4 and 5 only HHb and rCCO signals measured at 4 cm showed different responses to those of the extracerebral tissue. The clearest difference from the scalp response was observed at 4 cm in the rCCO response (Figures 4 and 5). No rCCO responses were observed at 1 cm and 3 cm using the homogeneous tissue model. Clear HHb-, tHB-, and rCCO-specific cerebral responses seen in Figure 7 and Table 2 indicate that the dynamics of changes measured at 3 cm and 4 cm channels were different from that measured at 1 cm, and this difference can be attributed to the differences between the brain and scalp responses to BHs. Note that hemodynamic responses at 3 cm and 4 cm shown in Figure 7 and Table 2 had significantly smaller magnitudes than those shown in Figures 4 and 5 and in Table 1. However, rCCO responses in both Figures 4 and 7 had their magnitudes close to 0.1 µM. This result supports the conclusion that we succeeded in decoupling rCCO changes from changes in other chromophores, and that the measured rCCO changes occurred in the brain. We would like to underline that in both homogeneous and two-layer algorithms we used the most conservative treatments of rCCO changes such as thresholding by the quantitative improvement in the goodness of fit, which suppressed spurious rCCO changes.

The time-courses of cerebral responses to BHs in healthy adult humans were studied in detail using blood-oxygen-level-dependent (BOLD) fMRI in [25,26]. The quantitative relationship between the BOLD changes measured by fMRI and hemodynamic signals measured by NIRS was investigated in [35]. Figure 8 (adopted from [25]) shows averaged BOLD signal time-courses with a 15 s BH after the full expiration on the areas supplied by the middle cerebral artery (MCA, red), anterior cerebral artery (ACA, blue) and posterior cerebral artery (PCA, black). Since our hNIRS probe was positioned on the left side of the forehead near the midline, it could interrogate cortical regions supplied by both ACA and MCA. The main difference between ACA and MCA regional responses was the early rise of the BOLD signal response in the ACA region and a 10 s delay in the MCA region. In our results the initial dynamics (during the first 15 s of BH) of cerebral HbO_2 and HHb responses rather corresponded to the MCA type of the BOLD response [25,33]. A delayed rCCO response after the regression (Figure 7) corresponded to the delayed ACA response. Such delayed cerebral responses were most different from the scalp hemodynamic responses to BHs measured at 1 cm (Figure 4), which were also very significant.

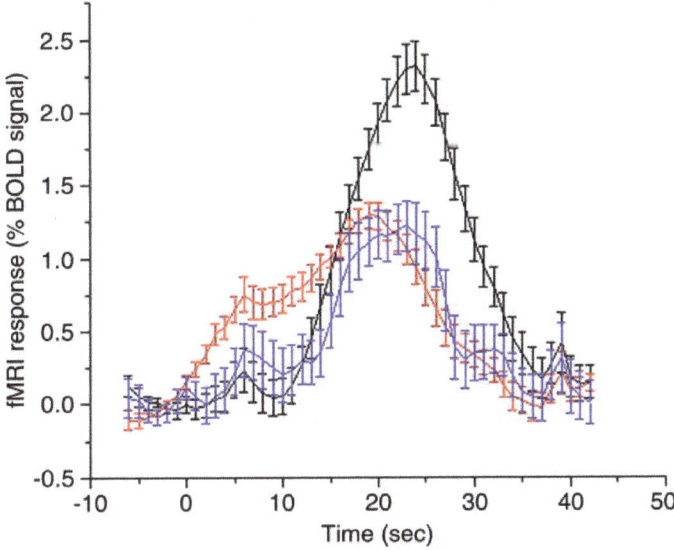

Figure 8. (Adapted from [23]) Averaged BOLD signal time-course with breath holding of 15 s after expiration on areas supplied by the MCA (red), ACA (blue), and PCA (black).

Another significant difference between the long- and short-distance channels was the longer peak times of HHb responses in the short-distance channel (longer than BH duration, Table 1). The peak times of responses to BHs after expiration measured by hNIRS at 4 cm were close to those measured by BOLD fMRI in [26] (see Figure 2 in [26]).

Our results show that without using a short-distance channel to remove biasing by the scalp, the cerebral responses to BHs were clearest in the rCCO time-course at 4 cm. Some features different from the scalp responses could also be seen in the HHb time-course at 4 cm. At 3 cm, some features of the cerebral response could be poorly recognized in the HHb time-course. The HbO_2 time-course did not show clear cerebral responses to BH at 3 cm or at 4 cm, in particular due to the high inter-subject variability. However, measurement of rCCO changes required hyperspectral or many-wavelength multispectral technology.

We found the waveband 750–900 nm be optimal for the detection of cerebral responses to BHs in adults. The wavelength that exhibited the largest fractional change in the detected optical signal with respect to the baseline value both at 3 and 4 cm was between 800 and 850 nm, which was in good agreement with the results of [13] (830 nm).

5. Conclusions

Cerebral changes could be efficiently separated from the extra-cerebral biasing using the time-domain linear regression of hNIRS signals measured at 3 cm and 4 cm source-detector separations by the signals from the short-distance channel. Without using the short-distance channel, none of the signals measured at 3 cm clearly reflected cerebral changes. At 4 cm source-detector separation, cerebral changes could be detected without using short-distance channels in the [HHb] and [rCCO] time-courses. The clearest cerebral responses were detected in the [rCCO] time-course at 4 cm. The optimal waveband for the rCCO measurements was between 750 nm and 900 nm. The [HbO_2] time-course at all source-detector distances was most dominated by the extracerebral biasing and therefore it was least suitable for cerebral signal detection. Further clinical studies are required to investigate the ability of the NIRS breath-holding paradigm to detect cerebral circulation disorders.

Author Contributions: Conceptualization, S.L. and V.T.; methodology, V.T.; software, V.T.; validation, S.L., V.T. and Z.G.; formal analysis, Z.G.; investigation, Z.G.; resources, V.T.; data curation, V.T.; writing—original draft preparation, V.T.; writing—review and editing, S.L.; visualization, Z.G.; supervision, V.T.; project administration, V.T.; funding acquisition, V.T. All authors have read and agreed to the published version of the manuscript.

Funding: This research received no external funding.

Institutional Review Board Statement: The study was conducted according to the guidelines of the Declaration of Helsinki, and approved by the Research Ethics Board of Ryerson University (REB: 2008-003-1, 4 May 2015).

Informed Consent Statement: Informed consent was obtained from all subjects involved in the study.

Acknowledgments: This research was supported by the Dean's Research Fund, Faculty of Science, Ryerson University.

Conflicts of Interest: The authors declare no conflict of interest.

References

1. Jöbsis, F. Noninvasive, infrared monitoring of cerebral and myocardial oxygen sufficiency and circulatory parameters. *Science* **1977**, *198*, 1264–1267. [CrossRef] [PubMed]
2. Green, D.W.; Kunst, G. Cerebral oximetry and its role in adult cardiac, non-cardiac surgery and resuscitation from cardiac arrest. *Anaesthesia* **2017**, *72*, 48–57. [CrossRef]
3. Okada, E.; Firbank, M.; Schweiger, M.; Arridge, S.R.; Cope, M.; Delpy, D.T. Theoretical and experimental investigation of near-infrared light propagation in a model of the adult head. *Appl. Opt.* **1997**, *36*, 21–31. [CrossRef] [PubMed]
4. Tachtsidis, I.; Scholkmann, F. False positives and false negatives in functional near-infrared spectroscopy: Issues, challenges, and the way forward. *Neurophotonics* **2016**, *3*, 039801. [CrossRef] [PubMed]
5. Wyser, D.; Mattille, M.; Wolf, M.; Lambercy, O.; Scholkmann, F.; Gassert, R. Short-channel regression in functional near-infrared spectroscopy is more effective when considering heterogeneous scalp hemodynamics. *Neurophotonics* **2020**, *7*, 035011. [CrossRef]
6. Milej, D.; Abdalmalak, A.; Rajaram, A.; St Lawrence, K. Direct assessment of extracerebral signal contamination on optical measurements of cerebral blood flow, oxygenation, and metabolism. *Neurophotonics* **2020**, *7*, 045002. [CrossRef] [PubMed]
7. Fantini, S.; Sassaroli, A. Frequency-domain techniques for cerebral and functional near-infrared spectroscopy. *Front. Neurosci.* **2020**, *14*, 300. [CrossRef]
8. Gregg, N.M.; White, B.R.; Zeff, B.W.; Berger, A.J.; Culver, J.P. Brain specificity of diffuse optical imaging: Improvements from superficial signal regression and tomography. *Front. Neuroenerg.* **2010**, *2*, 14. [CrossRef]
9. Gagnon, L.; Perdue, K.; Greve, D.N.; Goldenholz, D.; Kaskhedikar, G.; Boas, D.A. Improved recovery of the hemodynamic response in diffuse optical imaging using short optode separations and state-space modeling. *NeuroImage* **2011**, *56*, 1362–1371. [CrossRef]
10. Yücel, M.A.; Selb, J.; Aasted, C.M.; Petkov, M.P.; Becerra, L.; Borsook, D.; Boas, D.A. Short separation regression improves statistical significance and better localizes the hemodynamic response obtained by near-infrared spectroscopy for tasks with differing autonomic responses. *Neurophotonics* **2015**, *2*, 035005. [CrossRef]
11. Saager, R.B.; Berger, A.J. Direct characterization and removal of interfering absorption trends in two-layer turbid media. *J. Opt. Soc. Am. A* **2005**, *22*, 1874–1882. [CrossRef]
12. Brigadoi, S.; Cooper, R.J. How short is short? Optimum source–detector distance for short-separation channels in functional near-infrared spectroscopy. *Neurophotonics* **2015**, *2*, 025005. [CrossRef]

13. Cheng, X.; Sie, E.J.; Boas, D.A.; Marsili, F. Choosing an optimal wavelength to detect brain activity in functional near-infrared spectroscopy. *Opt. Lett.* **2021**, *46*, 924–927. [CrossRef] [PubMed]
14. Dunne, L.; Hebden, J.; Tachtsidis, I. Development of a near infrared multi-wavelength, multi-channel, time-resolved spec-trometer for measuring brain tissue haemodynamics and metabolism. *Adv. Exp. Med. Biol.* **2014**, *812*, 181–186, Erratum in *Adv. Exp. Med. Biol.* **2014**, *812*. [CrossRef]
15. Song, X.; Chen, X.; Chen, L.; An, X.; Ming, D. Performance Improvement for Detecting Brain Function Using fNIRS: A Multi-Distance Probe Configuration With PPL Method. *Front. Hum. Neurosci.* **2020**, *14*, 569508. [CrossRef]
16. Song, X.; Chen, X.; Wang, Z.; An, X.; Ming, D. MBLL with weighted partial path length for multi-distance probe configura-tion of fNIRS. In Proceedings of the 2019 41st Annual International Conference of the IEEE Engineering in Medicine and Biology Society (EMBC), Berlin, Germany, 23–27 July 2019; pp. 4766–4769. [CrossRef] [PubMed]
17. Giannoni, L.; Lange, F.; Tachtsidis, I. Hyperspectral imaging solutions for brain tissue metabolic and hemodynamic moni-toring: Past, current and future developments. *J. Opt.* **2018**, *20*, 044009. [CrossRef]
18. Bale, G.; Elwell, C.E.; Tachtsidis, I. From Jöbsis to the present day: A review of clinical near-infrared spectroscopy meas-urements of cerebral cytochrome-c-oxidase. *J. Biomed. Opt.* **2016**, *21*, 091307, Erratum in *J. Biomed. Opt.* **2016**, *21*. [CrossRef] [PubMed]
19. Heekeren, H.R.; Kohl, M.; Obrig, H.; Wenzel, R.; von Pannwitz, W.; Matcher, S.J.; Dirnagl, U.; Cooper, C.E.; Villringer, A. Noninvasive assessment of changes in cytochrome-c oxidase oxidation in human subjects during visual stimulation. *J. Cereb. Blood Flow Metabol.* **1999**, *19*, 592–603. [CrossRef]
20. Chan, S.T.; Ordway, C.; Calvanio, R.J.; Buonanno, F.S.; Rosen, B.R.; Kwong, K.K. Cerebrovascular Responses to O2-CO2 Exchange Ratio under Brief Breath-Hold Challenge in Patients with Chronic Mild Traumatic Brain Injury. *J. Neurotrauma* **2021**, *22*. [CrossRef] [PubMed]
21. McIntosh, R.C.; Hoshi, R.A.; Timpano, K.R. Take my breath away: Neural activation at breath-hold differentiates individuals with panic disorder from healthy controls. *Respir. Physiol. Neurobiol.* **2020**, *277*, 103427. [CrossRef]
22. Lin, W.; Xiong, L.; Han, J.; Leung, T.; Leung, H.; Chen, X.; Wong, K.S. Hemodynamic effect of external counterpulsation is a different measure of impaired cerebral autoregulation from vasoreactivity to breath-holding. *Eur. J. Neurol.* **2014**, *21*, 326–331. [CrossRef]
23. Schelkanova, I.; Toronov, V. Independent component analysis of broadband near-infrared spectroscopy data acquired on adult human head. *Biomed. Opt. Express* **2012**, *3*, 64–74. [CrossRef]
24. Holper, L.; Mann, J.J. Test–retest reliability of brain mitochondrial cytochrome-c-oxidase assessed by functional near-infrared spectroscopy. *J. Biomed. Opt.* **2018**, *23*, 056006. [CrossRef]
25. Leoni, R.F.; Mazzeto-Betti, K.C.; Andrade, K.C.; de Araujo, D.B. Quantitative evaluation of hemodynamic response after hypercapnia among different brain territories by fMRI. *Neuroimage* **2008**, *41*, 1192–1198. [CrossRef]
26. Pinto, J.; Bright, M.G.; Bulte, D.P.; Figueiredo, P. Cerebrovascular Reactivity Mapping without Gas Challenges: A Method-ological Guide. *Front. Physiol.* **2021**, *11*, 608475. [CrossRef] [PubMed]
27. Shrout, P.; Fleiss, J. Intraclass correlations: Uses in assessing rater reliability. *Psychol. Bull.* **1979**, *86*, 420–428. [CrossRef]
28. Toronov, V.; Franceschini, M.A.; Filiaci, M.; Fantini, S.; Wolf, M.; Michalos, A.; Gratton, E. Near-infrared study of fluctuations in cerebral hemodynamics during rest and motor stimulation: Temporal analysis and spatial mapping. *Med. Phys.* **2000**, *27*, 801–815. [CrossRef] [PubMed]
29. Ghali, M.G.Z.; Ghali, G.Z. Mechanisms Contributing to the Generation of Mayer Waves. *Front. Neurosci.* **2020**, *14*, 395. [CrossRef]
30. Yeganeh, H.; Toronov, V.; Elliott, J.; Diop, M.; Lee, T.; St. Lawrence, K. Broadband continuous-wave technique to measure baseline values and changes in the tissue chromophore concentrations. *Biomed. Opt. Express* **2012**, *3*, 2761. [CrossRef] [PubMed]
31. Nosrati, R.; Lin, S.; Ramadeen, A.; Monjazebi, D.; Dorian, P.; Toronov, V. Cerebral Hemodynamics and Metabolism During Cardiac Arrest and Cardiopulmonary Resuscitation Using Hyperspectral Near Infrared Spectroscopy. *Circ. J.* **2017**, *81*, 879–887. [CrossRef]
32. Fabbri, F.; Sassaroli, A.; Henry, M.E.; Fantini, S. Optical measurements of absorption changes in two-layered diffusive media. *Phys. Med. Biol.* **2004**, *49*, 1183. [CrossRef]
33. Baker, W.B.; Parthasarathy, A.B.; Ko, T.S.; Busch, D.R.; Abramson, K.; Tzeng, S.Y.; Mesquita, R.C.; Durduran, T.; Greenberg, J.H.; Kung, D.K.; et al. Pressure modulation algorithm to separate cerebral hemodynamic signals from extracerebral artifacts. *Neurophotonics* **2015**, *2*, 035004. [CrossRef]
34. Scholkmann, F.; Wolf, M. General equation for the differential pathlength factor of the frontal human head depending on wavelength and age. *J. Biomed. Opt.* **2013**, *18*, 105004. [CrossRef]
35. Toronov, V.; Walker, S.; Gupta, R.; Choi, J.H.; Gratton, E.; Hueber, D.; Webb, A. The roles of changes in deoxyhemoglobin concentration and regional cerebral blood volume in the fMRI BOLD signal. *Neuroimage* **2003**, *19*, 1521–1531. [CrossRef]

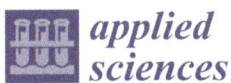

Article

Dual-Slope Diffuse Reflectance Instrument for Calibration-Free Broadband Spectroscopy

Giles Blaney *, Ryan Donaldson [†], Samee Mushtak [†], Han Nguyen [†], Lydia Vignale [†], Cristianne Fernandez, Thao Pham, Angelo Sassaroli and Sergio Fantini

Department of Biomedical Engineering, Tufts University, Medford, MA 02155, USA; Ryan.Donaldson@tufts.edu (R.D.); Samee.Mushtak@tufts.edu (S.M.); Han.Nguyen@tufts.edu (H.N.); Lydia.Vignale@tufts.edu (L.V.); Cristianne.Fernandez@tufts.edu (C.F.); Thao.Pham@tufts.edu (T.P.); Angelo.Sassaroli@tufts.edu (A.S.); sergio.fantini@tufts.edu (S.F.)
* Correspondence: Giles.Blaney@tufts.edu
† These authors contributed equally to this work.

Citation: Blaney, G.; Donaldson, R.; Mushtak, S.; Nguyen, H.; Vignale, L.; Fernandez, C.; Sassaroli, A.; Pham, T.; Fantini, S. Dual-Slope Diffuse Reflectance Instrument for Calibration-Free Broadband Spectroscopy. *Appl. Sci.* **2021**, *11*, 1757. https://doi.org/10.3390/app11041757

Academic Editor: Johannes Kiefer

Received: 29 December 2020
Accepted: 12 February 2021
Published: 16 February 2021

Publisher's Note: MDPI stays neutral with regard to jurisdictional claims in published maps and institutional affiliations.

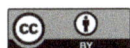

Copyright: © 2021 by the authors. Licensee MDPI, Basel, Switzerland. This article is an open access article distributed under the terms and conditions of the Creative Commons Attribution (CC BY) license (https:// creativecommons.org/licenses/by/ 4.0/).

Abstract: This work presents the design and validation of an instrument for dual-slope broadband diffuse reflectance spectroscopy. This instrument affords calibration-free, continuous-wave measurements of broadband absorbance of optically diffusive media, which may be translated into absolute absorption spectra by adding frequency-domain measurements of scattering at two wavelengths. An experiment on a strongly scattering liquid phantom (milk, water, dyes) confirms the instrument's ability to correctly identify spectral features and measure absolute absorption. This is done by sequentially adding three dyes, each featuring a distinct spectral absorption, to the milk/water phantom. After each dye addition, the absorption spectrum is measured, and it is found to reproduce the spectral features of the added dye. Additionally, the absorption spectrum is compared to the absorption values measured with a commercial frequency-domain instrument at two wavelengths. The measured absorption of the milk/water phantom quantitatively agrees with the known water absorption spectrum ($R^2 = 0.98$), and the measured absorption of the milk/water/dyes phantom quantitatively agrees with the absorption measured with the frequency-domain instrument in six of eight cases. Additionally, the measured absorption spectrum correctly recovers the concentration of one dye, black India ink, for which we could accurately determine the extinction spectrum (i.e., the specific absorption per unit concentration). The instrumental methods presented in this work can find applications in quantitative spectroscopy of optically diffusive media, and particularly in near-infrared spectroscopy of biological tissue.

Keywords: broadband diffuse reflectance spectroscopy; frequency-domain near-infrared spectroscopy; dual-slope; absorption spectra

1. Introduction

Diffuse optics is concerned with the propagation of light in highly-scattering or diffusive media. One notable application is Near-Infrared Spectroscopy (NIRS) of biological tissue, which is typically performed in the wavelength range from about 600 nm to about 1000 nm [1–3]. Diffuse optics finds a variety of applications in several fields of study. In food science [4], it may be applied for inspection [5] or evaluation [6]. In pharmaceutical manufacturing, diffuse optics may join other process analytical technologies, for example to analyze and characterize particles [7] or powders [8]. A few other examples include archaeological soil analysis [9], dendrology (study of wood) [10], and art authentication analysis [11]. In the study of biological tissue, diffuse optics finds applications in basic research, medical diagnostics, and physiological monitoring. Examples include clinical brain monitoring [12], the study of brain activation [13], breast imaging [14], and muscle measurements in sports science [15]. This is by no means an exhaustive list. The work that we present in this article aims to improve the accuracy and robustness of quantitative broadband spectroscopy of optically turbid media, and it is relevant to a variety of applications of diffuse optics, even though we mostly focus on its role in the area of biomedical optics.

Quantitatively, light propagation in diffusive media is characterized by a lower probability of absorption (related to the absorption coefficient; μ_a) compared to the probability of effectively isotropic scattering (related to the reduced scattering coefficient; μ_s'). These two optical properties are the chief quantities of interest in the field of diffuse optics and diffuse biomedical optics [2,3,16,17], and they feature a wavelength dependence that is often of crucial importance. In the case of most biological tissues, the dominating scattering condition of diffuse optics is realized in the NIR optical window. Measurements of the wavelength dependent absorption of tissue yields information about the concentration of chromophores with known extinction spectra, while measurements of scattering spectra yields structural information related to the size and density of scattering centers [2].

These properties are often obtained in the reflectance geometry, where light is delivered onto the sample surface and detected at some distance away from the source on the same surface. The primary difficulty in these measurements is the decoupling of absorption and scattering contributions to the measured optical signal. One method to achieve this is by using a source light with a temporally varying intensity. These time-resolved methods fall into two categories: time-domain methods where the light emission has an impulse profile, and Frequency-Domain (FD) methods where the light emission has a sinusoidal profile [1,18]. Focusing on FD-NIRS, the measurement of both absorption and scattering can be achieved via a calibrated measurement of the spatial dependence (as a function of the distance from the source on the tissue surface) of the amplitude and phase of the detected modulated intensity (which may be represented as a complex reflectance) [19–21].

This spatially dependent measurement of FD-NIRS data to achieve absolute optical properties is often summarized as measuring the slope (versus source-detector distance; ρ) of a modified intensity amplitude and phase (i.e., modified complex reflectance). The chief complication of this technique is calibration, since each source-detector pair may have differing instrumental contributions (because of the individual source emission and detector sensitivity properties) and differing coupling factors between source/detector and sample. A method which compensates for the differing instrumental contributions is the so-called Multi-Distance (MD) scanning, where either the source or the detector is moved across the surface of the optical medium [22]. In doing so, the instrumental factors remain the same for each distance (same source and same detector used for each distance); thus, the measurement of slope is independent of these factors. However, differing coupling factors may still be present if during the scan the source (or detector) moves away or toward the tissue surface (in a non-contact case), or experiences a variable contact pressure (in a contact case). Aside from MD scanning, a potentially more effective and more easily implemented calibration free method may be employed. This method is the Self-Calibrating (SC) method, where a symmetric optical probe that features two sources and two detectors is used such that instrumental and coupling factors cancel in the calculation of slopes [23]. This method is also effective at suppressing motion artifacts [24] and allows calibration-free saturation measurements with Continuous-Wave (CW) methods after assuming the wavelength dependence of scattering [25]. The original purpose of the SC method was to achieve measurements of absolute optical properties with FD-NIRS. However, recently the optode geometry inspired by the SC method has been extended to the use of only the amplitude or phase of the complex reflectance in FD-NIRS [26,27]. This extension was named Dual-Slope (DS) since it relies on the average of two slopes measured with this special optode configuration.

One of the limitations of time-resolved NIRS methods, such as FD-NIRS, is the added instrumental complexity compared to CW. There has been work in broadband time-resolved spectroscopy [28]; however, such instruments require complex instruments (super-continuum lasers, single photon counting, and instrument response calibration).

Because of this, the norm in time-resolved NIRS methods is the use of two or a few wavelengths as opposed to a continuous broadband spectrum [1]. In contrast, CW methods may use White-Light or broadband light sources, such as halogen lamps, and spectrometer detectors, since there is no need for measurements of fast temporal characteristics. These spectroscopic methods in CW are so-called Diffuse Reflectance Spectroscopy (DRS) due to their collection geometry and use of a spectrometer as a detector (instead of avalanche photodiodes or photomultiplier tubes typical in time-resolved methods). Therefore, CW broadband DRS (CW-bDRS) has the advantage of collecting data over many wavelengths but the disadvantage that absorption and scattering are coupled and inseparable due to the use of CW illumination. A solution that has become more and more common is to combine a time-resolved NIRS instrument at few wavelengths with a CW-bDRS system [29–34]. Such a technique allows extrapolation of scattering from few to many wavelengths, by assuming a power law decay of the reduced scattering coefficient with wavelength [2], as well as decoupling of absorption from scattering in the CW-bDRS data.

At this point, a small note on nomenclature is valuable. The acronym MD FD-NIRS refers to a frequency-domain method capable of measuring absolute optical properties (absorption and scattering) at discrete wavelengths from measurements at multiple distances between source and detector. The acronym CW-bDRS refers to a continuous-wave technique capable of measuring wavelength-resolved data (which depends on absorption and scattering) over a range of many wavelengths. Further, to achieve a calibration free full spectral technique, DS CW-bDRS is introduced. It is noted that the distinction between SC (self-calibrating) and DS (dual-slope) is the use of complex reflectance in SC FD-NIRS versus continuous-wave reflectance in DS CW-bDRS, for example. The main focus of this work will be to develop the DS CW-bDRS technique in combination with MD FD-NIRS to decouple absorption and scattering contributions to the absorbance spectra.

In this paper, a new DS CW-bDRS/MD FD-NIRS instrument is described and validated by measuring absolute absorption spectra of highly scattering media, or phantoms. The novelty of this work is the design of a CW instrument for broadband spectroscopy that implements DS methods for robust and calibration free measurements of absorbance spectra. The addition of MD FD-NIRS measurements at two wavelengths allows for the translation of absorbance spectra into quantitative absorption spectra. The organization of the paper is as follows. The methods, in Section 2, are split into techniques, in Section 2.1, where FD-NIRS and CW-bDRS are described, and is followed by experiments, Section 2.2, which lays out a phantom experiment, and then by an analysis, Section 2.3, which explains methods to calculate optical properties. Next, the results, Section 3, report measured phantom absorption spectra. Finally, the discussion, Section 4, elaborates on the validation of the DS CW-bDRS/MD FD-NIRS instrument.

2. Materials and Methods

2.1. Techniques

2.1.1. Frequency-Domain Near-Infrared Spectroscopy

Frequency-Domain Near-Infrared Spectroscopy (FD-NIRS) was implemented with the purpose of measuring absolute optical properties of highly scattering media. Those being the absorption coefficient (μ_a) and the reduced scattering coefficient (μ_s'). A commercial FD-NIRS instrument was used (Imagent V2, ISS, Champaign, IL, USA) operating with a modulation frequency of 140.625 MHz and optical wavelengths of 690 and 830 nm.

FD-NIRS was implemented in a Multi-Distance scan (MD FD-NIRS). To achieve this, a single detector fiber bundle ($\varnothing$3 mm) was held at a fixed location and two co-localized source fibers ($\varnothing$600 µm; two wavelengths) were scanned via a linear stage (Figure 1a). In doing so, the complex reflectance (amplitude and phase) was measured at eleven distances (from 15 to 25 mm spaced by 1 mm; Figure 1b). This MD scan allowed for measurements of complex reflectance slopes (amplitude and phase) versus source-detector distance without the need for calibration (assuming unchanging coupling with the sample since the same fibers are used for each distance and the fiber/sample contact remains about the same during the linear scan). These measurements were used to calculate the absolute optical properties of the diffuse medium as described in Section 2.3.

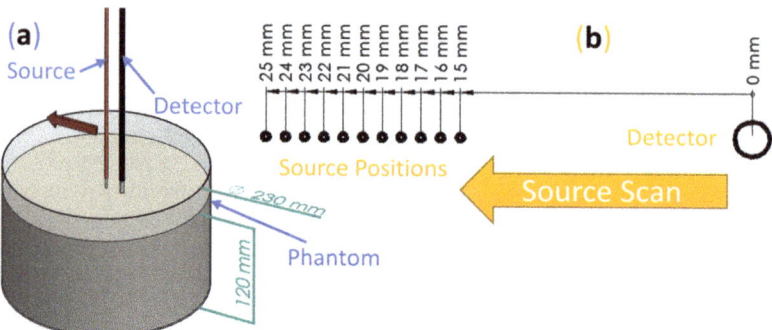

Figure 1. Frequency-domain near-infrared spectroscopy methods to achieve measurements of absolute optical properties. (a) Render of multi-distance scan done on diffuse optical phantoms. (b) Schematic of eleven different source positions realized during the multi-distance scan.

2.1.2. Broadband Diffuse Reflectance Spectroscopy

Continuous-Wave broadband Diffuse Reflectance Spectroscopy (CW-bDRS) was implemented with the purpose of measuring absolute absorption spectra of optically diffusive media (Figure 2a). This was realized using a Dual-Slope (DS) optode geometry which allowed for calibration free measurements of the CW reflectance slope (versus source-detector distance). The DS optode configuration (Figure 2c) used was the same as described previously [26]; it contains two source positions and two detector positions. The linearly symmetric arrangement resulted in a calibrated measurement of the slope (versus source-detector distance) of CW reflectance from 25 to 35 mm.

The DS CW-bDRS system was custom built to achieve the multiplexing needed for DS measurements. This measurement requires the reflectance signal be acquired from all combinations of sources (named 1 and 2) and detectors (named A and B; Figure 2c). To do so, both the sources and detectors must be multiplexed (Figure 2b). Sources were multiplexed by using two shuttered light sources (AvaLight-HAL-S-Mini, Avantes, Louisville, CO, USA), each connected to one source position. Shutter state was controlled via a Transistor-Transistor Logic (TTL) signal from a micro-controller (Uno R3, Arduino, Ivrea, Italy) which was connected to the control computer via Universal Serial Bus (USB). Light was delivered from the sources to the probe using ⌀2 mm fiber bundles. The light sources output an approximate black-body spectrum with a temperature of about 2650 K (peak at about 1000 nm). On the detector side, diffuse CW light was collected using a ⌀600 μm fiber at each of the two detector positions. Multiplexing of the detector positions was done using a 1 × 2 fiber switch (LBMB, Photonwares, Woburn, MA, USA) where the common end was connected to a spectrometer (AvaSpec-HERO, Avantes) via a ⌀600 μm fiber. The spectrometer was configured with a 500 μm slit and collected 1024 wavelengths between about 498 nm and about 1064 nm.

The bottleneck in the multiplexing sequence is the switching time of the fiber switch. Because of this, the cycle of source-detector position combinations was optimized to minimize fiber switch actuation. Naming source-detector combinations as source number (1 or 2), then detector letter (A or B; Figure 2c) as an example measurement sequence could be:

$$\ldots 1A] \to [1A \diamond 2A \blacktriangleright 2B \diamond 1B] \to [1B \diamond 2B \blacktriangleright 2A \diamond 1A] \to [1A \ldots$$

where "⋄" is a source switch, "▶" is a detector switch, and the square brackets show one full DS set acquisition. The reflectance from each source-detector combination is linearly interpolated to the average absolute time for their corresponding DS set. The four reflectance measurements that contribute to a DS measurement are synchronous, thus preventing potential temporal artifacts when studying dynamic samples or biological tissue. The specific acquisition parameters (including sampling rate and wavelength range considered) are stated in Section 2.2, and the analysis of the DS data (slope of CW reflectance versus source-detector distance) to yield absolute absorption spectra is described in Section 2.3.

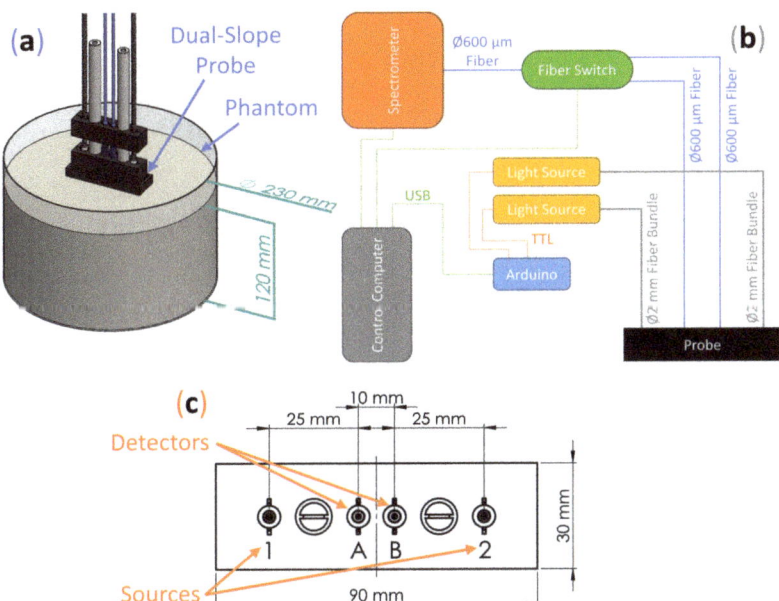

Figure 2. Broadband diffuse reflectance spectroscopy methods to achieve measurements of absolute absorption spectra. (**a**) Render of diffuse reflectance spectroscopy probe on a diffuse optical phantom. (**b**) Schematic of dual-slope diffuse reflectance spectroscopy device. Acronyms: Universal Serial Bus (USB) and Transistor-Transistor Logic (TTL). (**c**) Schematic of the source (1 and 2) and detector (A and B) positions on the dual-slope diffuse reflectance spectroscopy probe.

2.2. Experiment

The purpose of the experiment was to validate the Dual-Slope broadband Diffuse Reflectance Spectroscopy (DS CW-bDRS) instrument. This was done using a liquid optical phantom which was measured at different dyes concentrations to confirm the DS CW-bDRS's ability to distinguish spectral features and measure absolute absorption. A total of 5 L of the phantom was made and placed in a cylindrical tank (Figures 1a and 2a). The base of the phantom was made of 2% (reduced fat) Milk and Water (MW; 43% milk and 57% water volume fraction) such that the scattering properties were similar to those of biological tissue in the near-infrared. The scattering was assumed to not change as dyes were added since the addition of the dyes is expected to have a negligible effect on scattering. Each time the phantom was measured, the measurement was done by both Multi-Distance Frequency-Domain Near-Infrared Spectroscopy (MD FD-NIRS) and DS CW-bDRS.

Three dyes were added in the following order: black India-Ink (II; Higgins, Leeds, MA, USA), NIR746A (N7; QCR Solutions, Palm City, FL, USA), and NIR869A (N8; QCR Solutions). II is expected to have a relatively flat or decreasing absorption spectrum with wavelength in the Near-Infrared (NIR) range [35,36]. By contrast, N7 and N8 are expected to have absorption peaks at around 746 nm and 869 nm, respectively (Figure 3). However, the actual peak wavelength may shift depending on the chemical properties of the solvent [37,38].

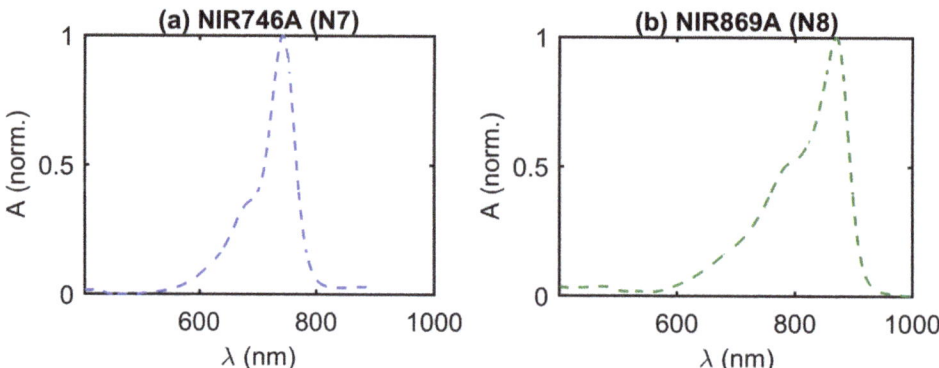

Figure 3. Expected spectral features of near-infrared dyes in water, provided by the manufacturer (QCR Solutions, Palm City, FL, USA). [37] (**a**) Normalized Absorbance (A) versus wavelength (λ) of NIR746A dye (N7). (**b**) Normalized A of NIR869A dye (N8).

The measurements and dye additions proceeded as follows (measurements meaning both MD FD-NIRS and DS CW-bDRS). First, the MW base phantom was mixed, then measured. Then, II was mixed in and the phantom measured again. Next, N7 was mixed and again the phantom measured. Finally, N8 was also mixed into the phantom and the measurement was done for a final time. The amount of each addition of dye was such that all absorption spectra were expected to stay within typical absorption values of biological tissue (approximately 0.005 to 0.020 mm^{-1}) [2].

The temporal sampling parameters of the DS CW-bDRS system were set to yield a relatively fast sampling rate while still measuring a relevant wavelength range. Along these lines, DS CW-bDRS data were analyzed between 600 nm and 900 nm and the sampling rate was set to 2.5 Hz. For DS CW-bDRS 5 min of data were averaged for analysis. The MD FD-NIRS measurement took 30 s at each step for a total measurement time of 5.5 min (eleven steps; Section 2.1.1), and had a sampling rate of 2.8 Hz. These parameters were chosen such that the rate and time of DS CW-bDRS and MD FD-NIRS were approximately equal.

This phantom experiment resulted in MD FD-NIRS measurements at two wavelengths and DS CW-bDRS measurements between 600 nm and 900 nm for four phantoms (MW, MW+II, MW+II+N7, and MW+II+N7+N8). Section 2.3 describes the analysis of these data to result in absolute optical properties at two wavelengths and absolute absorption spectra.

2.3. Analysis

In Section 2.1, two techniques were described: Multi-Distance Frequency-Domain Near-Infrared Spectroscopy (MD FD-NIRS; Section 2.1.1) and Dual-Slope Continuous-Wave broadband Diffuse Reflectance Spectroscopy (DS CW-bDRS; Section 2.1.2). MD yields the spatial dependence of reflectance across multiple distances, while DS yields two symmetric spatial dependencies of reflectance. Additionally, FD-NIRS yields complex reflectance (at a few wavelengths), while CW-bDRS yields CW reflectance (at many wavelengths). However, regardless of these differences, the same basic analysis was used to find absolute optical properties (with the process repeated for each separate wavelength). In the following, we first describe the analysis of complex reflectance across multiple distances (MD FD-NIRS). Then, we explain how the method is modified to handle DS data and what additional assumptions are needed to use CW data (DS CW-bDRS).

Considering a semi-infinite medium with extrapolated-boundary conditions, the complex reflectance ($\widetilde{R}$), defined as the net optical flux exiting the tissue per unit source power, may be written as [2,39]:

$$\widetilde{R} = \frac{1}{4\pi}\left(\widetilde{C_1}e^{-\widetilde{\mu}_{eff}r_1} + \widetilde{C_2}e^{-\widetilde{\mu}_{eff}r_2}\right), \tag{1}$$

$$\widetilde{C_1} = z_0 \left(\frac{1 + \widetilde{\mu_{eff}} r_1}{r_1^3} \right) \quad \widetilde{C_2} = -z_0' \left(\frac{1 + \widetilde{\mu_{eff}} r_2}{r_2^3} \right), \tag{2}$$

$$r_1 = \sqrt{\rho^2 + z_0^2} \quad r_2 = \sqrt{\rho^2 + z_0'^2}, \tag{3}$$

where z_0 is the depth of the real isotropic source ($z_0 = 1/\mu_s'$), z_0' is the height of the imaginary isotropic source ($z_0' = -z_0 + 2z_b$), ρ is the source-detector distance on the surface of the semi-infinite medium, and $\widetilde{\mu_{eff}}$ is the complex effective attenuation coefficient. The extrapolated boundary height ($z_b = 2A/(3(\mu_s' + \mu_a))$) and the complex effective attenuation coefficient ($\widetilde{\mu_{eff}} = \sqrt{3(\mu_s' + \mu_a)(\mu_a - \omega n_{in} i/c)}$) are both expressed in terms of the absorption coefficient (μ_a), reduced scattering coefficient (μ_s'). The remaining parameters are the angular modulation frequency (ω), the reflection parameter (A), the index of refraction inside the medium (n_{in}; assumed to be 1.4, typical for biological tissue [2]), and the speed of light in vacuum (c). Additionally, $\omega = 2\pi f_{mod}$, where f_{mod} is the modulation frequency. Finally, A is a function of n_{in} and the index of refraction outside the medium (n_{out}; assumed to be 1.0) [39]. To yield a linear relationship, Equation (1) can be rewritten as:

$$\ln\left[\frac{4\pi \widetilde{R}}{\widetilde{C_1} + \widetilde{C_2} e^{\widetilde{\mu_{eff}}(r_1 - r_2)}}\right] = -\widetilde{\mu_{eff}} r_1, \tag{4}$$

which shows a linear dependence of a modified complex reflectance ($\widetilde{y} = \ln[4\pi \widetilde{R}/(\widetilde{C_1} + \widetilde{C_2} e^{\widetilde{\mu_{eff}}(r_1 - r_2)})]$) on r_1 (i.e., $\widetilde{y} = -\widetilde{\mu_{eff}} r_1$).

The linear complex slope ($-\widetilde{\mu_{eff}}$) in Equation (4) is used to calculate the desired optical properties (μ_a and μ_s'). However, $\widetilde{y}$ is dependent on μ_a and μ_s', and r_1 is dependent on μ_s'. Thus, an iterative method is used to recover the $\widetilde{\mu_{eff}}$:

$$\widetilde{y}[\mu_{a,k}, \mu_{s,k}'] = -\widetilde{\mu_{eff}}_{k+1} r_1[\mu_{s,k}'] + \widetilde{b}_{k+1}, \tag{5}$$

where k is the iteration number, and $\widetilde{b}$ is the complex intercept (dependent on instrumental factors not considered in Equation (4)). For the iterative method, an initial guess of μ_a and μ_s' is needed for $k = 0$. This guess was determined based on the linear slopes of complex reflectance amplitude and phase as previously described [19,21]. At each iteration, the current values of $\widetilde{y}$ and r_1 were used to fit a complex linear slope ($-\widetilde{\mu_{eff}}$):

$$\begin{bmatrix} -\widetilde{\mu_{eff}} \\ \widetilde{b} \end{bmatrix}_{k+1} = \begin{bmatrix} r_{1,1} & 1 \\ \vdots & \vdots \\ r_{1,n} & 1 \end{bmatrix}_k^+ \begin{bmatrix} \widetilde{y}_1 \\ \vdots \\ \widetilde{y}_n \end{bmatrix}_k, \tag{6}$$

where the + superscript is the Moore-Penrose inverse, $\widetilde{b}$ is the complex intercept (ignored), and there are n measurements (distances). In the case of MD FD-NIRS, $n = 11$ since there were eleven measurements of complex reflectance at eleven different source-detector distances. To convert $\widetilde{\mu_{eff}}$ to μ_a and μ_s' the following expressions were used:

$$\mu_t' = \frac{-2c\Re\left[\widetilde{\mu_{eff}}\right]\Im\left[\widetilde{\mu_{eff}}\right]}{3n\omega}, \tag{7}$$

$$\mu_a = \frac{\Re\left[\widetilde{\mu_{eff}}\right]^2 - \Im\left[\widetilde{\mu_{eff}}\right]^2}{3\mu_t'}, \tag{8}$$

where μ_t' is the total reduced attenuation coefficient, and $\mu_s' = \mu_t' - \mu_a$. At each iteration, the new fitted $-\widetilde{\mu_{eff}}$ yielded the μ_a and μ_s' used to calculate $\widetilde{y}$ and r_1 for the next iteration (Equation (5)). The procedure terminated when the condition $|\widetilde{\mu_{eff}}_k - \widetilde{\mu_{eff}}_{k-1}| < 10^{-4}$ L/mm was met.

The above expressions show how MD FD-NIRS data were used to find absolute μ_a and μ_s' at two wavelengths. To extend this to DS CW-bDRS, first, Equation (6) was modified to use DS data. DS yields two symmetric measurements of R versus ρ (where R is now real not complex since CW data is used). Thus, instead of Equation (6), the following was used for DS CW-bDRS:

$$\mu_{eff_{k+1}} = \frac{-1}{2}\left(\frac{y_{2,1} - y_{1,1}}{r_{1,2,1} - r_{1,1,1}} + \frac{y_{2,2} - y_{1,2}}{r_{1,2,2} - r_{1,1,2}}\right)_k, \qquad (9)$$

where the first subscript of y and second subscript of r_1 corresponds to source-detector distance, and the second and third subscript, respectively, corresponds to the symmetric slope in the DS set. This expression is simply the average of the slopes of y versus r_1 between the two DS symmetric sets. In addition, note that the tildes were removed since y is now real (from real R). This results in a real effective attenuation coefficient ($\mu_{eff} = \sqrt{3\mu_a(\mu_s' + \mu_a)}$) instead of a complex one. Equations (1)–(5) may all be used as is, with removing the tilde hats to now represent real data.

Since the DS CW-bDRS method yields a real μ_{eff}, μ_s' must be known to find μ_a using the following expression instead of Equation (8):

$$\mu_a = \sqrt{\frac{\mu_s'^2}{4} + \frac{\mu_{eff}^2}{3}} - \frac{\mu_s'}{2}. \qquad (10)$$

To address the need to know μ_s', the data from the MD FD-NIRS measurements were used. FD-NIRS yielded a measurement of μ_s' at two wavelengths ($\mu_{s,FD}'(\lambda_1)$ and $\mu_{s,FD}'(\lambda_2)$; where λ is wavelength). These μ_s' measurements are then extrapolated using the following expression to find μ_s' at all the wavelengths used by bDRS:

$$\mu_s'(\lambda) = \mu_{s,FD}'(\lambda_1)\left(\frac{\lambda}{\lambda_1}\right)^{\frac{-\ln[\mu_{s,FD}'(\lambda_2)/\mu_{s,FD}'(\lambda_1)]}{\ln[\lambda_1/\lambda_2]}}. \qquad (11)$$

Therefore, when analyzing DS CW-bDRS data, μ_a is found for each wavelength using the assumed μ_s' expressed above for each wavelength.

In summary, the same basic method, based on iteratively fitting to Equation (4), is used for MD FD-NIRS and DS CW-bDRS to find absolute optical properties. DS differs from MD in the calculation of slope, and the μ_s' from MD FD-NIRS is extrapolated to find an assumed μ_s' for each DS CW-bDRS wavelength.

3. Results

The phantom experiment described in Section 2.2 consisted of measuring four phantoms, each with both Multi-Distance Frequency-Domain Near-Infrared Spectroscopy (MD FD-NIRS; Figure 1a) and Dual-Slope Continuous Wave broadband Diffuse Reflectance Spectroscopy (DS CW-bDRS; Figure 2a). The phantoms were Milk and Water (MW), that with India Ink added (MW+II), then that again with NIR746A added (MW+II+N7), and then that yet again with NIR869A added (MW+II+N7+N8).

Figure 4 shows the results of this experiment. The absolute absorption (μ_a) spectrum is shown across wavelengths (λ) for all four phantoms and two measurement methods (Figure 4a). Additionally, Figure 4a shows a dashed line representing the modeled (as 99.1% water [40,41] and 0.9% lipid [42] volume fractions) absorption of the MW phantom. The coefficient of determination (R^2) was calculated for the MW data and model, yielding a value of 0.98, implying that 98% of the variance in the MW data is explained by the modeled MW absorption. In Figure 4b–d, the change in absorption ($\Delta\mu_a$) as a result of adding the three different dyes (II, N7, and N8) is shown. The error regions in all plots are dominated by the systematic uncertainty in the distances on the DS-CW-bDRS probe (estimated at ±0.1 mm for chained dimensions) and within the MD-FD-NIRS measurement (estimated at ±0.5 mm for initial position and ±0.01 mm for scan pitch). Note the flat absorption contribution from II and the spectral features from N7 and N8. Particularly, a peak between 700 nm and 800 nm for N7 and a peak between 800 nm and 900 nm for N8. How these results serve to validate the instrument will be discussed in Section 4. Briefly, notice the agreement between the MD FD-NIRS and DS CW-bDRS measurements and the agreement between the expected MW spectrum and the DS CW-bDRS measured MW spectrum.

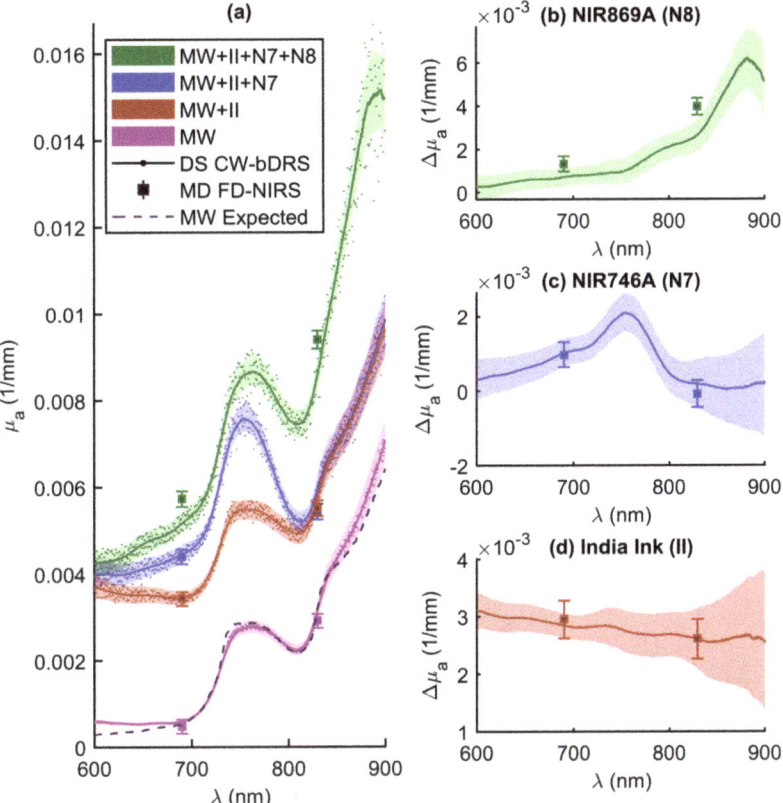

Figure 4. Results from phantom experiment. (**a**) Absolute absorption (μ_a) spectra as a function of wavelength (λ). Showing results from Dual-Slope Continuous-Wave broadband Diffuse Reflectance Spectroscopy (DS CW-bDRS) and Multi-Distance Frequency-Domain Near-Infrared Spectroscopy (MD FD-NIRS) measurements. Spectra shown for the following phantoms: Milk and Water (MW), MW plus India Ink (II), MW plus II plus NIR746A (N7), and, finally, MW plus II plus N7 plus NIR869A (N8). DS CW-bDRS points show individual wavelength measurements and lines show smoothed (moving average) spectra for visualization. Dashed line shows the expected spectrum for MW modeled as water and lipid. (**b**) Change in absorption ($\Delta \mu_a$) from adding N8 (i.e., $\mu_a^{MW+II+N7+N8} - \mu_a^{MW+II+N7}$), (**c**) $\Delta \mu_a$ from adding N7 (i.e., $\mu_a^{MW+N7} - \mu_a^{MW+II}$), and (**d**) $\Delta \mu_a$ from adding II (i.e., $\mu_a^{MW+II} - \mu_a^{MW}$).

4. Discussion

The experiment involved a liquid phantom and sought to validate the Dual-Slope Continuous Wave broadband Diffuse Reflectance Spectroscopy (DS CW-bDRS) instrument (Sections 2.2 and 3). This was done by measuring a highly scattering phantom as dyes were progressively added (Figure 4). The expectation was that the DS CW-bDRS (in combination with Multi-Distance Frequency-Domain Near-Infrared Spectroscopy; MD FD-NIRS) instrument would be able to measure the known spectral features of the dyes and the absolute absorption of the phantom.

First, before any dyes were added (just Milk and Water; MW), the phantom was measured to yield an absorption spectrum dominated by water (Figure 4a). This MW spectra had the expected spectral features of water (hump at about 750 nm and sharp increase starting at about 800 nm) [41]. Further, the expected MW spectrum agrees (within error) with the experimental data for the spectral range between 690 nm and 830 nm, where the reduced scattering coefficient is interpolated (not extrapolated) from the MD FD-NIRS measurement. Below 690 nm, the agreement is lost likely due to the very low water absorption, such that, even low absorption, contributions from fat, proteins, or other milk constituents in the MW medium may become detectable. Above 830 nm, the agreement also degrades possibly because of incorrect reduced scattering values (from extrapolation) or contributions from other absorbers in the milk other than water. Overall, the quantitative agreement between the expected and measured MW spectra are quite good with a coefficient of determination (R^2) of 0.98, indicating an accurate measurement of absolute absorption by DS CW-bDRS.

Further, the absorption measured by MD FD-NIRS agrees within error with DS CW-bDRS at all points of comparison except for NIR869A (N8). For N8, the difference between the measurements is about 10%, and the combined errors for the two measurements amount to about 8% (dominated by uncertainty in the distances; Section 3). Admittedly, the reduced scattering found by MD FD-NIRS is used to find the absorption for DS CW-bDRS; thus, the measurements are related (Section 2.3). However, the observed agreement demonstrates a reliable absolute measurement of the slope of diffuse reflectance with the DS CW-bDRS instrument, given the accurate measurements with the scanning MD method used by MD FD-NIRS in controlled laboratory conditions. In the case of N8, where the two instruments do not agree, the most likely explanation is instrumental error (distance uncertainty and boundary conditions). The distance uncertainty accounts for most of the difference between the measurements, and the remaining unaccounted disagreement may be explained by uncertainties in boundary conditions (true depth of fibers in phantom, existence of meniscus, etc.). These distance uncertainties and boundary effects may have changed for each measurement, since after the addition of each dye the instruments needed to be re-setup and placed on the phantom. This may explain why instrumental errors impacted differently the measurements of different dyes. Additionally, there is evidence that the NIR dyes are not stable over time (discussed below), and the two measurements are not simultaneous (5–10 min between measurements). Any of these considerations may have led to the lack of agreement for N8. However, given the existence of these considerations and the close agreement in six out of eight cases, we find that the results serves to validate the absolute absorbance measured by DS CW-bDRS.

Focusing on the individual dye additions allows for validation of the measurement of spectral features. The first dye added was India Ink (II), which is expected to have a flat or decreasing spectral dependence with wavelength [35]. The change in the absorption spectrum observed confirmed this wavelength dependence and, again, agreed with the measurements at two wavelengths with MD FD-NIRS (Figure 4d). Further evaluation was carried out to estimate the recovered concentration of II given the measured change in absorption. The true concentration (in volume fraction) of II in the phantom was 5.7×10^{-6}, given the phantom volume and the amount of ink added. The same II was measured in transmission in non-diffuse solutions of known concentrations to yield spectra of the total attenuation coefficient (μ_t; assuming only unscattered light is detected). To yield the spectrum of absorption (μ_a; needed to recover concentration in the diffuse experiment) for II, the single scattering albedo (a) must be assumed ($\mu_a = \mu_t(1-a)$). This must be considered for II since it is not in solution in water but instead a suspension of carbon particles. Wavelength independent values of $a = 0$ to $a = 0.15$ were assumed which yielded recovered concentrations of 5.2×10^{-6} to 6.1×10^{-6}, respectively. This range of low albedo values of pure II indicates that its scattering coefficient is much smaller than the absorption coefficient, which is consistent with the literature [35,36]. The range resulted in measurement errors of -8.8% to 7.0% (given true value of 5.7×10^{-6}). Therefore, it is expected that DS CW-bDRS is capable of recovering accurate chromophore concentrations given that the extinction spectra is known (not the case here since the albedo for II was not measured). For NIR746A (N7) and N8, the concentration recovery was not carried out due to temporal and spectral instability of the dyes (discussed below). Future experiments will be undertaken to validate the accurate chromophore concentration recovery of DS CW-bDRS using soluble and stable dyes.

Moving on from II, the next two dyes were expected to feature a more interesting spectrum (Figure 3). NIR746A (N7) was added after II and the change of absorption presented in Figure 4c. The expected peak between 700 nm and 800 nm was present. However, upon closer examination, the exact peak location is shifted about 12 nm higher for the DS CW-bDRS measurement compared to the expected spectrum (Figure 5a). When the next and final dye, NIR869A (N8), was added, yet again there was a peak present in approximately the expected location (Figure 4b). But, as with N7, there was an approximate 12-nm shift to longer wavelengths in the DS CW-bDRS measurement. This is consistent with a bathochromic shift, which is possible for these dyes given the manufacturer information and previous studies [37,38]. The hypothesis is that, when in milk, the dyes exhibit a bathochromic shift due to the different bulk polar nature of milk versus water. To test this possibility, two further measurements were done on N8. N8 was measured in transmission (in a semi-micro cuvette), both in water and in the MW mixture (Figure 5b). The results show that the transmission spectral absorbance for N8 in milk matches the DS CW-bDRS peak location, whereas the transmission spectral absorbance of N8 in water matches the manufacturer provided spectra. Thus, this transmission experiment supports the hypothesis that these dyes exhibit a bathochromic shift of about 12 nm when in the MW mixture. However, it is unknown if the amplitude of the absorption peak is also effected (hyperchromic or hypochromic shift) for these dyes. The dyes were also found to be temporally unstable, as extended time in solution caused N7 to lose its near-infrared absorption peak, and N8's peak shifted roughly 200 nm to the blue. These spectral and temporal instabilities stopped the analysis of the concentrations of these dyes in the diffuse phantom. But, despite this, DS CW-bDRS was still capable of distinguishing the dye's spectral features.

Summarizing the discussion above, these results on the liquid phantom serve to validate the DS CW-bDRS instrument's ability to measure spectral features and absolute values of absorption in a diffuse medium. In six of eight cases (all except 690 nm and 830 nm for N8), the absolute absorption measured with DS CW-bDRS agreed within error with MD FD-NIRS. DS CW-bDRS also accurately measured the expected absorption spectrum of MW ($R^2 = 0.98$). Additionally, the DS CW-bDRS instrument correctly measured the flat spectra of II and the peaks of N7 and N8. The concentration of II was estimated, suggesting the ability to recover chromophore concentrations given the extinction. Finally, it was confirmed that the recovered peak locations of the N7 and N8 dyes are what is expected for these dyes in milk. Future work will be done to validate the overall methods ability to accurately recover chromophore concentrations.

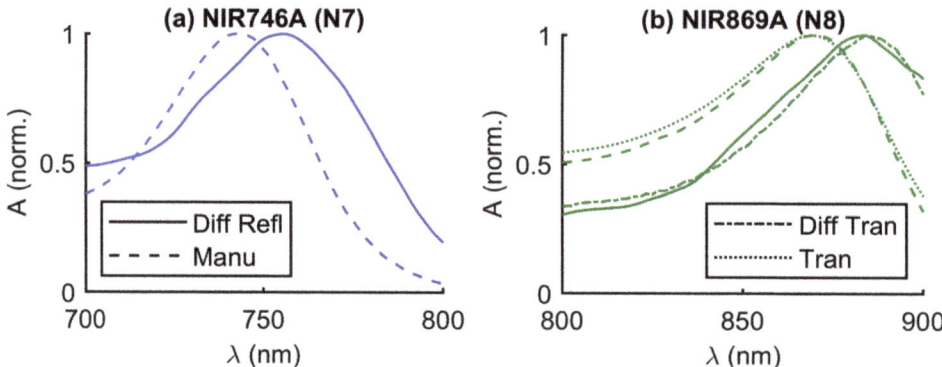

Figure 5. Comparison of wavelength (λ) normalized Absorbance (A) peak locations for two dyes. Four types of spectra shown: Diffuse Reflectance (Diff Refl, i.e., in milk), provided by the Manufacturer (Manu; (QCR Solutions, Palm City FL, USA) [37], i.e., in water), Diffuse Transmission (Diff Tran, i.e., in milk), and Transmission (Tran, i.e., in water). (**a**) NIR746A (N7) dye. (**b**) NIR869A (N8) dye.

5. Conclusions

In this article, we have presented a new Dual-Slope Continuous Wave broadband Diffuse Reflectance Spectroscopy (DS CW-bDRS) instrument. Experiments on highly scattering liquid phantoms demonstrated the instrument's capability of measuring absolute absorbance spectra without any need for instrumental calibration. By combining DS CW-bDRS and Frequency-Domain Near-Infrared Spectroscopy (FD-NIRS; to account for scattering contributions to the absorbance spectrum), we were able to measure absolute absorption spectra of the liquid phantoms that contained a combination of three dyes. These experiments demonstrated the technique's ability to perform absolute spectral absorption measurements and retrieve the correct spectral features of various dyes. Future work will focus on further validation of chromophore concentration measurements. The importance of this work lies in the development of the DS CW-bDRS instrument. This DS CW-bDRS instrument is novel in that it combines DS and bDRS to achieve calibration-free measurements and provides a valuable tool for absolute spectral measurements of highly scattering media, including biological tissues.

Author Contributions: Conceptualization, G.B. and S.F.; methodology, G.B., R.D., S.M., H.N., L.V., C.F., A.S., T.P., and S.F.; software, G.B., R.D., S.M., H.N., and L.V.; validation, G.B., R.D., S.M., H.N., L.V., and C.F.; formal analysis, G.B.; investigation, G.B., R.D., S.M., H.N., L.V., and C.F.; resources, A.S. and S.F.; data curation, G.B., A.S., and S.F.; writing—original draft preparation, G.B., A.S., and S.F.; writing—review and editing, G.B., C.F., A.S., T.P., and S.F.; visualization, G.B.; supervision, G.B., C.F., A.S., and S.F.; project administration, G.B. and S.F.; funding acquisition, S.F. All authors have read and agreed to the published version of the manuscript.

Funding: This work was funded by the National Institutes of Health (NIH) grant R01 NS095334.

Data Availability Statement: Data and supporting codes are available upon request.

Conflicts of Interest: The authors declare no conflict of interest. The funders had no role in the design of the study; in the collection, analyses, or interpretation of data; in the writing of the manuscript, or in the decision to publish the results.

References

1. Fantini, S.; Sassaroli, A. Frequency-Domain Techniques for Cerebral and Functional Near-Infrared Spectroscopy. *Front. Neurosci.* **2020**, *14*, 1–18. [CrossRef] [PubMed]
2. Bigio, I.J.; Fantini, S. *Quantitative Biomedical Optics*; Cambridge University Press: Cambridge, UK, 2016.
3. Scholkmann, F.; Kleiser, S.; Metz, A.J.; Zimmermann, R.; Mata Pavia, J.; Wolf, U.; Wolf, M. A review on continuous wave functional near-infrared spectroscopy and imaging instrumentation and methodology. *NeuroImage* **2014**, *85*, 6–27. [CrossRef]

4. Ozaki, Y.; McClure, W.F.; Christy, A.A. *Near-Infrared Spectroscopy in Food Science and Technology*; John Wiley & Sons: Hoboken, NJ, USA, 2006.
5. Johnson, J.B. An overview of near-infrared spectroscopy (NIRS) for the detection of insect pests in stored grains. *J. Stored Prod. Res.* **2020**, *86*, 101558. [CrossRef]
6. Kademi, H.I.; Ulusoy, B.H.; Hecer, C. Applications of miniaturized and portable near infrared spectroscopy (NIRS) for inspection and control of meat and meat products. *Food Rev. Int.* **2019**, *35*, 201–220. [CrossRef]
7. Razuc, M.; Grafia, A.; Gallo, L.; Ramírez-Rigo, M.V.; Romañach, R.J. Near-infrared spectroscopic applications in pharmaceutical particle technology. *Drug Dev. Ind. Pharm.* **2019**, *45*, 1565–1589. [CrossRef]
8. Stranzinger, S.; Markl, D.; Khinast, J.G.; Paudel, A. Review of sensing technologies for measuring powder density variations during pharmaceutical solid dosage form manufacturing. *TrAC Trends Anal. Chem.* **2020**, 116147. [CrossRef]
9. Trant, P.L.K.; Kristiansen, S.M.; Sindbæk, S.M. Visible near-infrared spectroscopy as an aid for archaeological interpretation. *Archaeol. Anthropol. Sci.* **2020**, *12*, 280. [CrossRef]
10. Tsuchikawa, S.; Kobori, H. A review of recent application of near infrared spectroscopy to wood science and technology. *J. Wood Sci.* **2015**, *61*, 213–220. [CrossRef]
11. Chen, Z.; Gu, A.; Zhang, X.; Zhang, Z. Authentication and inference of seal stamps on Chinese traditional painting by using multivariate classification and near-infrared spectroscopy. *Chemom. Intell. Lab. Syst.* **2017**, *171*, 226–233. [CrossRef]
12. Lange, F.; Tachtsidis, I. Clinical Brain Monitoring with Time Domain NIRS: A Review and Future Perspectives. *Appl. Sci.* **2019**, *9*, 1612. [CrossRef]
13. Agbangla, N.F.; Audiffren, M.; Albinet, C.T. Use of near-infrared spectroscopy in the investigation of brain activation during cognitive aging: A systematic review of an emerging area of research. *Ageing Res. Rev.* **2017**, *38*, 52–66. [CrossRef] [PubMed]
14. Grosenick, D.; Rinneberg, H.; Cubeddu, R.; Taroni, P. Review of optical breast imaging and spectroscopy. *J. Biomed. Opt.* **2016**, *21*, 091311. [CrossRef] [PubMed]
15. Perrey, S.; Ferrari, M. Muscle Oximetry in Sports Science: A Systematic Review. *Sport. Med.* **2018**, *48*, 597–616. [CrossRef]
16. Durduran, T.; Choe, R.; Baker, W.B.; Yodh, A.G. Diffuse optics for tissue monitoring and tomography. *Rep. Prog. Phys.* **2010**, *73*, 076701. [CrossRef]
17. Jacques, S.L.; Pogue, B.W. Tutorial on diffuse light transport. *J. Biomed. Opt.* **2008**, *13*, 041302. [CrossRef]
18. Fishkin, J.B.; Gratton, E. Propagation of photon-density waves in strongly scattering media containing an absorbing semi-infinite plane bounded by a straight edge. *J. Opt. Soc. Am. A* **1993**, *10*, 127. [CrossRef]
19. Blaney, G.; Sassaroli, A.; Pham, T.; Krishnamurthy, N.; Fantini, S. Multi-Distance Frequency-Domain Optical Measurements of Coherent Cerebral Hemodynamics. *Photonics* **2019**, *6*, 83. [CrossRef]
20. Hallacoglu, B.; Sassaroli, A.; Guerrero-Berroa, E.; Schnaider Beeri, M.; Haroutunian, V.; Shaul, M.; Rosenberg, I.H.; Toren, A.; Fantini, S. Absolute measurement of cerebral optical coefficients, hemoglobin concentration and oxygen saturation in old and young adults with near-infrared spectroscopy. *J. Biomed. Opt.* **2012**, *17*, 081406. [CrossRef] [PubMed]
21. Fantini, S.; Hueber, D.; Franceschini, M.A.; Gratton, E.; Rosenfeld, W.; Stubblefield, P.G.; Maulik, D.; Stankovic, M.R. Non-invasive optical monitoring of the newborn piglet brain using continuous-wave and frequency-domain spectroscopy. *Phys. Med. Biol.* **1999**, *44*, 1543–1563. [CrossRef]
22. Fantini, S.; Franceschini, M.A.; Gratton, E. Semi-infinite-geometry boundary problem for light migration in highly scattering media: A frequency-domain study in the diffusion approximation. *JOSA B* **1994**, *11*, 2128–2138. [CrossRef]
23. Hueber, D.M.; Fantini, S.; Cerussi, A.E.; Barbieri, B.B. New optical probe designs for absolute (self-calibrating) NIR tissue hemoglobin measurements. In *Optical Tomography and Spectroscopy of Tissue III*; International Society for Optics and Photonics: San Jose, CA, USA, 1999; Volume 3597, pp. 618–631. [CrossRef]
24. Scholkmann, F.; Metz, A.J.; Wolf, M. Measuring tissue hemodynamics and oxygenation by continuous-wave functional near-infrared spectroscopy—How robust are the different calculation methods against movement artifacts? *Physiol. Meas.* **2014**, *35*, 717–734. [CrossRef] [PubMed]
25. Kleiser, S.; Ostojic, D.; Nasseri, N. In vivo precision assessment of a near-infrared spectroscopy-based tissue oximeter (OxyPrem v1.3) in neonates considering systemic hemodynamic fluctuations. *J. Biomed. Opt.* **2018**, *23*, 1. [CrossRef]
26. Blaney, G.; Sassaroli, A.; Pham, T.; Fernandez, C.; Fantini, S. Phase dual-slopes in frequency-domain near-infrared spectroscopy for enhanced sensitivity to brain tissue: First applications to human subjects. *J. Biophotonics* **2020**, *13*. [CrossRef]
27. Sassaroli, A.; Blaney, G.; Fantini, S. Dual-slope method for enhanced depth sensitivity in diffuse optical spectroscopy. *J. Opt. Soc. Am. A* **2019**, *36*, 1743. [CrossRef]
28. Lanka, P.; Segala, A.; Farina, A.; Konugolu Venkata Sekar, S.; Nisoli, E.; Valerio, A.; Taroni, P.; Cubeddu, R.; Pifferi, A. Non-invasive investigation of adipose tissue by time domain diffuse optical spectroscopy. *Biomed. Opt. Express* **2020**, *11*, 2779. [CrossRef]
29. Vasudevan, S.; Forghani, F.; Campbell, C.; Bedford, S.; O'Sullivan, T.D. Method for quantitative broadband diffuse optical spectroscopy of tumor-like inclusions. *Appl. Sci.* **2020**, *10*, 1419. [CrossRef]
30. Ganesan, G.; Warren, R.V.; Leproux, A.; Compton, M.; Cutler, K.; Wittkopp, S.; Tran, G.; O'Sullivan, T.; Malik, S.; Galassetti, P.R.; et al. Diffuse optical spectroscopic imaging of subcutaneous adipose tissue metabolic changes during weight loss. *Int. J. Obes.* **2016**, *40*, 1292–1300. [CrossRef] [PubMed]

31. Konugolu Venkata Sekar, S.; Dalla Mora, A.; Bargigia, I.; Martinenghi, E.; Lindner, C.; Farzam, P.; Pagliazzi, M.; Durduran, T.; Taroni, P.; Pifferi, A.; et al. Broadband (600–1350 nm) Time-Resolved Diffuse Optical Spectrometer for Clinical Use. *IEEE J. Sel. Top. Quantum Electron.* **2016**, *22*, 406–414. [CrossRef]
32. O'Sullivan, T.D.; Cerussi, A.E.; Cuccia, D.J.; Tromberg, B.J. Diffuse optical imaging using spatially and temporally modulated light. *J. Biomed. Opt.* **2012**, *17*, 0713111. [CrossRef]
33. Tachtsidis, I.; Gao, L.; Leung, T.S.; Kohl-Bareis, M.; Cooper, C.E.; Elwell, C.E. A Hybrid Multi-Distance Phase and Broadband Spatially Resolved Spectrometer and Algorithm for Resolving Absolute Concentrations of Chromophores in the Near-Infrared Light Spectrum. In *Oxygen Transport to Tissue XXXI, Advances in Experimental Medicine and Biology*; Springer: Boston, MA, USA, 2010; pp. 169–175. [CrossRef]
34. Bevilacqua, F.; Berger, A.J.; Cerussi, A.E.; Jakubowski, D.; Tromberg, B.J. Broadband absorption spectroscopy in turbid media by combined frequency-domain and steady-state methods. *Appl. Opt.* **2000**, *39*, 6498. [CrossRef]
35. Di Ninni, P.; Martelli, F.; Zaccanti, G. The use of India ink in tissue-simulating phantoms. *Opt. Express* **2010**, *18*, 26854. [CrossRef] [PubMed]
36. Martelli, F.; Zaccanti, G. Calibration of scattering and absorption properties of a liquid diffusive medium at NIR wavelengths. CW method. *Opt. Express* **2007**, *15*, 486–500. [CrossRef] [PubMed]
37. Water Soluble NIR Dyes—QCR Solutions Corp. Available online: https://qcrsolutions.com/water-soluble-near-infrared-dyes/ (accessed on 1 June 2020).
38. Cugmas, B.; Naglič, P.; Menachery, S.P.M.; Pernuš, F.; Likar, B. Poor optical stability of molecular dyes when used as absorbers in water-based tissue-simulating phantoms. In *Design and Quality for Biomedical Technologies XII*; Liang, R., Hwang, J., Eds.; SPIE: San Francisco, CA, USA, 2019; Volume 10870, pp. 56–65. [CrossRef]
39. Contini, D.; Martelli, F.; Zaccanti, G. Photon migration through a turbid slab described by a model based on diffusion approximation. I. Theory. *Appl. Opt.* **1997**, *36*, 4587–4599. [CrossRef] [PubMed]
40. Pope, R.M.; Fry, E.S. Absorption spectrum (380–700 nm) of pure water II Integrating cavity measurements. *Appl. Opt.* **1997**, *36*, 8710. [CrossRef] [PubMed]
41. Kou, L.; Labrie, D.; Chylek, P. Refractive indices of water and ice in the 065- to 25-mum spectral range. *Appl. Opt.* **1993**, *32*, 3531. [CrossRef] [PubMed]
42. van Veen, R.; Sterenborg, H.; Pifferi, A.; Torricelli, A.; Cubeddu, R. Determination of VIS- NIR absorption coefficients of mammalian fat, with time- and spatially resolved diffuse reflectance and transmission spectroscopy. In *Biomedical Topical Meeting*; OSA: Washington, DC, USA, 2004; p. SF4. [CrossRef]

Article

Comparison of Optical Imaging Techniques to Quantitatively Assess the Perfusion of the Gastric Conduit during Oesophagectomy

Maxime D. Slooter [1], Sanne M. A. Jansen [2], Paul R. Bloemen [2], Richard M. van den Elzen [2], Leah S. Wilk [2], Ton G. van Leeuwen [2], Mark I. van Berge Henegouwen [1,*], Daniel M. de Bruin [2] and Suzanne S. Gisbertz [1]

1 Department of Surgery, Cancer Center Amsterdam, Amsterdam UMC, University of Amsterdam, 1105 AZ Amsterdam, The Netherlands; m.d.slooter@amsterdamumc.nl (M.D.S.); s.s.gisbertz@amsterdamumc.nl (S.S.G.)
2 Department of Biomedical Engineering & Physics, Cancer Center Amsterdam, Amsterdam Cardiovascular Sciences, Amsterdam UMC, University of Amsterdam, 1105 AZ Amsterdam, The Netherlands; sma.jansen@hotmail.com (S.M.A.J.); p.r.bloemen@amsterdamumc.nl (P.R.B.); r.m.vandenelzen@amsterdamumc.nl (R.M.v.d.E.); l.s.wilk@amsterdamumc.nl (L.S.W.); t.g.vanleeuwen@amsterdamumc.nl (T.G.v.L.); d.m.debruin@amsterdamumc.nl (D.M.d.B.)
* Correspondence: m.i.vanbergehenegouwen@amsterdamumc.nl

Received: 5 July 2020; Accepted: 5 August 2020; Published: 10 August 2020

Abstract: In this study, four optical techniques—Optical Coherence Tomography, Sidestream Darkfield Microscopy, Laser Speckle Contrast Imaging, and Fluorescence Angiography (FA)—were compared on performing an intraoperative quantitative perfusion assessment of the gastric conduit during oesophagectomy. We hypothesised that the quantitative parameters show decreased perfusion towards the fundus in the gastric conduit and in patients with anastomotic leakage. In a prospective study in patients undergoing oesophagectomy with gastric conduit reconstruction, measurements were taken with all four optical techniques at four locations from the base towards the fundus in the gastric conduit (Loc1, Loc2, Loc3, Loc4). The primary outcome included 14 quantitative parameters and the anastomotic leakage rate. Imaging was performed in 22 patients during oesophagectomy. Ten out of 14 quantitative parameters significantly indicated a reduced perfusion towards the fundus of the gastric conduit. Anastomotic leakage occurred in 4/22 patients (18.4%). At Loc4, the FA quantitative values for "$T_{1/2}$" and "mean slope" differed between patients with and without anastomotic leakage ($p = 0.025$ and $p = 0.041$, respectively). A quantitative perfusion assessment during oesophagectomy is feasible using optical imaging techniques, of which FA is the most promising for future research.

Keywords: optical imaging; fluorescence imaging; fluorescence angiography; indocyanine green (ICG); optical coherence tomography (OCT); laser speckle contrast imaging (LSCI); esophagectomy; gastric conduit; Sidestream Darkfield Microscopy (SDF); multispectral

1. Introduction

Surgical morbidity related to inadequate perfusion is a major challenge after oesophagectomy with gastric conduit reconstruction for oesophageal cancer. This type of surgical morbidity includes anastomotic leakage and graft necrosis, and remains high even after recent developments in minimally invasive surgery, enhanced recovery programs, and the centralisation of cancer surgery, occurring in up to 20% of the patients [1–4].

To achieve digestive continuity after oesophagectomy, the replacement of the native oesophagus by a constructed gastric conduit is a potential solution. The perfusion of the gastric conduit is mainly based on the right gastroepiploic artery, which usually terminates before the future anastomotic site, causing the future anastomotic site to be at risk for inadequate perfusion. Surgeons assess the perfusion of the gastric conduit by observing the colour of the serosal surface, the bleeding of resection margins, or arterial palpation. To aid surgeons' decision-making, different optical imaging techniques have been introduced to assess perfusion intraoperatively [5,6].

Optical imaging, which is established by the interaction between light and tissue, is potentially able to image changes in perfusion real-time and at high resolution. These characteristics of optical imaging have the potential to analyse a perfusion intraoperatively and in a quantitative manner [7,8]. Some optical imaging techniques are already Food and Drug Administration (FDA)-approved and Conformité Européenne (CE)-marked systems, but others lack clinical evaluation [5,9]. Not all techniques have an adequate specificity for patient outcomes and are so far unable to objectify perfusion in quantitative values for clinical usage [5]. The comparison of techniques in the literature is hampered by the large range of available imaging systems and the heterogeneity of quantitative parameters and perfusion endpoints [5]. Therefore, there is scant evidence on which optical imaging technique and related quantitative parameter is the most predictive for inadequate perfusion and patient outcomes.

In this explorative study (IDEAL phase 2a), we aim to compare four optical techniques using different wavelengths of light on performing a quantitative perfusion assessment of the gastric conduit in patients undergoing oesophagectomy with gastric conduit reconstruction for oesophageal cancer. The four optical techniques are Optical Coherence Tomography (OCT), Sidestream Darkfield Microscopy (SDF), Laser Speckle Contrast Imaging (LSCI), and Fluorescence Angiography (FA). We hypothesised that the quantitative parameters of the optical techniques show decreased perfusion (A) towards the fundus in the gastric conduit and (B) in patients with anastomotic leakage. By comparing these four techniques, we aimed for a recommendation of an optical imaging technique for a quantitative perfusion assessment of the gastric conduit for future studies and clinical intraoperative use.

2. Materials and Methods

2.1. Study

This is a single-centre, prospective, observational study in patients undergoing elective oesophagectomy with gastric conduit reconstruction for oesophageal cancer. This study adhered to the STARD (Standards for Reporting of Diagnostic Accuracy Studies) [10] and STROBE (STrengthening the Reporting of OBservational studies in Epidemiology) [11] guidelines.

This study was approved by the Institutional Review Board of the Amsterdam UMC, location AMC, (NL52377.018.15) and submitted to the clinicaltrials.gov database (NCT02902549) [12]. Written informed consent was obtained from all patients.

2.2. Procedure

All the procedures were performed totally minimally invasively with laparoscopy and thoracoscopy. A McKeown (cervical anastomosis) or Ivor Lewis (intrathoracic anastomosis) procedure was performed by two specialised upper-gastrointestinal surgeons (MIvBH, SSG), as previously described [13]. The stomach was reconstructed into a 3–4 cm wide gastric conduit using a powered linear stapler. Directly after gastric conduit reconstruction, perfusion measurements were performed using four optical techniques in the following order: OCT, SDF, LSCI, and FA. Perfusion measurements were performed at four locations (Loc1–4): 3 cm proximal of the level of (Loc1), at the level of (Loc2), 3 cm distal to (Loc3) at the level of the watershed between the right and left gastroepiploic artery, and at the level of the gastric fundus (Loc4) (Figure 1). A sterile gauze was placed to point out the watershed area (the end of the right gastroepiploic artery). Subsequently, a cervical or intrathoracic anastomosis to the proximal oesophagus was constructed. The anastomotic site of the gastric conduit was determined by a conventional white light assessment, independent of imaging outcomes, and was located between Loc3 and Loc4.

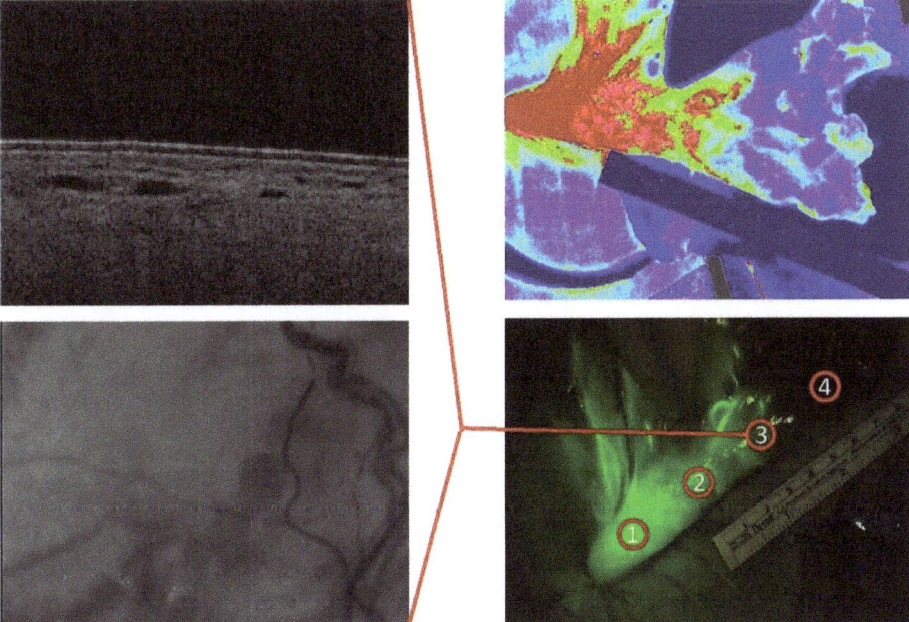

Figure 1. Qualitative images by all four imaging techniques: upper left Optical Coherence Tomography (OCT), lower left Sidestream Darkfield Imaging (SDF), upper right Laser Speckle Contrast Imaging (LSCI), and lower right Fluorescence Angiography (FA). Perfusion measurements were performed at four locations (Loc1–4): 3 cm proximal of the level of (Loc1), at the level of (Loc2), 3 cm distal to (Loc3) the level of the watershed between the right and left gastroepiploic artery, and at the level of the gastric fundus (Loc4).

2.3. Imaging Modalities and Software

OCT was performed by a commercial 50 kHz IVS 2000 swept source system (Santec, 5823 Ohkusa-Nenjozaka, Komaki-City, Aichi, Japan), an FDA-approved and CE-marked system, using a centre wavelength of ~1300 nm. Measurements were performed as previously described [14]. Data analysis was performed using custom-made scripts written in MATLAB (Mathworks, Natick, MA, USA) [14].

SDF is a hand-held, in-contact, green light (530 nm) imaging system that visualises microcirculation. Image contrast is based on the absorption of green light by oxyhaemoglobin in red blood cells (RBCs) [15]. Therefore, RBCs will appear as dark spots in the image. SDF measurements were performed by the Microscan (Microvision Medical, Amsterdam, The Netherlands), an FDA-approved system to monitor the microcirculation of critically ill patients. To stabilise the image, a custom-made stabiliser based on the design by Balestra et al. [16] was used to adhere the tissue to the imaging system. The SDF obtained images were analysed using the AVA3.2 software (Microvision Medical BV, Amsterdam, The Netherlands).

LSCI is a near infrared imaging system with a laser operating at 785 nm and measures speckle fluctuations induced by the motion and change in number of RBCs. The LSCI was used as previously described [17]. Imaging was performed by the MoorFLPI-1™ (Moor instruments, Devon, UK), an FDA-approved and CE-marked system, positioned at 40 cm above the gastric conduit, as measured by a laser distance meter (Leica Geosystems D110, Leica Camera, Wetzlar, Germany).

FA is a near infrared imaging modality that images the spatial distribution of the contrast agent indocyanine green (ICG), detecting at an emission wavelength of approximately 800 nm. FA was performed by the Artemis system® (Quest Medical Imaging, Middenmeer, The Netherlands), an FDA-approved and CE-marked system, after the intravenous administration of 2.5 mg of ICG. The Artemis system was placed under a 90-degree angle and also at a distance of 40 cm above the gastric conduit, as measured with the laser distance meter. A metric ruler was placed in the field of view for image calibration. The anaesthesiologist administered 2.5 mg of ICG intravenously. The perfusion was imaged in continuous video recordings of 2–3 min. In-house software was developed to plot the ICG in- and outflow in a fluorescence–time curve. A ruler in the field of view was used for calibration, and for every location a circular region of interest (ROI) with a diameter of 1 cm was used to measure the ICG signal.

2.4. Outcomes

The primary objective of this study was the comparison of the ability of the four optical imaging systems—OCT, SDF, LSCI, and FA—to obtain the quantitative perfusion parameters during surgery, and to explore the relation between the four locations (Loc1–4) and the occurrence of anastomotic leakage. The primary outcome included 14 quantitative parameters outlined below in "quantitative parameters" at four locations and anastomotic leakage. Quantitative assessment was deemed successful per technique when one or more measurements could be obtained per patient. Anastomotic leakage was defined by the Esophageal Complications Consensus Group (ECCG) classification and diagnosed by a CT-scan with contrast, upper gastrointestinal endoscopy, drainage of saliva, gastric content via wound/drains, and/or by reoperation [18].

The secondary outcomes were imaging characteristics and hemodynamic parameters. The imaging characteristics included the field of view, imaging depth, ease of use, practical limitations (overall and for quantitative analysis), invasiveness, time consumption, and quality. The quality was deemed high when no technical issues occurred to obtain qualitative images. The relations between the quantitative and hemodynamic parameters were explored at Loc1. Hemodynamic parameters were recorded at the start of imaging and included the mean arterial pressure (MAP; mmHg), heart rate (beats/min), systolic and diastolic blood pressure (mmHg), temperature nasopharynx (°C), cardiac output (L/min), stroke volume (mL), stroke volume variation (%), and cardiac index (L/min/m^2).

2.5. Quantitative Parameters

Fourteen quantitative parameters were measured (OCT $n = 1$, SDF $n = 6$, LSCI $n = 2$, and FA $n = 5$). The quantitative parameter for OCT was [14]:

1. The percentage of speckle contrast pixels (speckle %) indicative of the flow obtained in the M-mode of the scans;

Quantitative parameters derived for SDF included [15]:

2. Total vessel density (TVD): ratio between the total vessel length and the area of ROI (mm/mm^2);
3. Perfused vessel density (PVD): ratio between the perfused scored vessel length and the area of ROI (mm/mm^2);
4. Microvascular flow index (MFI): sum of the qualitative determination (0 no, 1 intermittent, 2 sluggish, 3 continuous) of the predominate flow in four quadrants of the SDF image, divided by four;
5. De Backer Score (DBS): number of vessels crossing a grid overlay divided by the total length of the vessels;
6. Proportion of perfused vessels (PPV): perfused vessel length divided by the total vessel length of the ROI in %;
7. Velocity (μm/s): assessed per selected vessels by a space–time diagram;

The quantitative parameters calculated for LSCI were [17]:

8. Flux in laser speckle perfusion units (LSPU);
9. Δ%Flux defined as the percentage difference in Flux relative to Loc1 (positive number when there is a decrease in Flux);

FA was quantified by the assessment of the time-dependent change in the fluorescence signal at the ROIs in the form of the software-derived fluorescence–time curves [8,19]. The quantitative parameters for FA included:

10. Influx time point (τ): time in seconds between the occurrence of the peak fluorescence in the right gastroepiploic artery and the time point at which the fluorescence intensity in the ROI was statistically significantly larger than the background;
11. F_{max}: maximal intensity in arbitrary units (AU) within 50 s after the influx time point. Fmax was corrected by subtracting the median background value measured from the start of imaging to the influx time point (τ);
12. T_{max}: time in seconds after the influx time point (τ) at which the background-corrected fluorescence intensity reached Fmax, also known as the time-to-peak;
13. $T_{1/2}$: time in seconds after the influx time point (τ) at which the background-corrected fluorescence intensity was half of the Fmax;
14. Mean slope: rate at which the fluorescence intensity increased (AU/s).

2.6. Statistics

The quantitative perfusion parameters were shown as the median and interquartile (IQR) or total range. All the available data were used for the analysis. The comparison of quantitative perfusion parameters between Loc1 and Loc4 were analysed using the Wilcoxon Signed Ranks Test. The results at Loc3 and Loc4 were compared between patients with or without anastomotic leakage using the Mann–Whitney U test. A p-value of below 0.05 was considered significant. Correlations between the quantitative values and hemodynamic parameters were assessed by calculating the Spearman's rank correlation coefficient ρ. A p-value ≤ 0.05 was considered statistically significant. The imaging characteristics were summarised using simple descriptive statistics or in quantitative terms. The added surgical time was shown in the median and IQR. All the analyses were performed using IBM® SPSS® Statistics (version 26.0.0, IBM Corporation, NY, USA).

3. Results

Between October 2015 and June 2016, in total 26 patients that underwent minimally invasive oesophagectomy with gastric conduit reconstruction were included after written informed consent was obtained. Four patients did not receive imaging due to extended operation time and were not taken into the analysis. The baseline characteristics of 22 patients are shown in Table 1 [17]. The gastric conduit was connected to the proximal oesophagus by a cervical ($n = 2$) or intrathoracic ($n = 20$) anastomosis.

Table 1. Baseline characteristics.

	Cohort ($n = 22$)
Age (years) median total range	62 (37–79)
Gender (male), n (%)	19 (86.4)
Body mass index (kg/m^2), median total range	25.9 (17.0–34.2)
Surgical procedures, n (%)	
Ivor Lewis	20 (91)
McKeown	2 (9)
Cardiovascular disease, n (%)	5 (23)
Diabetes Mellitus *, n (%)	2 (9)
COPD, n (%)	2 (9)

* Only diabetes mellitus type 2. COPD = chronic obstructive pulmonary disease.

3.1. Imaging Characteristics

Qualitative imaging was successful in all the patients ($n = 22$) with all four techniques. In Figure 1, qualitative images by all four imaging techniques are shown for one patient. The imaging characteristics are shown in Table 2. OCT and SDF had a narrow field of view, of which SDF assessed the microvasculature for a region of 1 mm × 1 mm. LSCI and FA were wide field techniques and showed similarity in the qualitative images (Figure 1). All the practical limitations are summarised in Table 2, of which artefacts, shadowing, and focus were limitations for quantitative analysis. The motion artefacts for OCT and SDF were secondary to the respiratory rate, heart rate, peristalsis, or probe handling, and other artefacts were due to air bubbles in the surgical drape. The use of OCT, SDF, LSCI, and FA added 6 (5–7), 5 (4–7), 3 (2–4), and 4 (2–4) minutes to the surgical time, respectively.

Table 2. Imaging characteristics.

	Field of View	Depth-Resolving	Ease of Use	Real-Time	Practical Limitations
OCT	10 mm × 10 mm × 2.5 mm	+	Sterile sheet, probe handling	+	Motion artefacts, shadowing
SDF	1 mm × 1 mm	-	Sterile sheet, tissue-contact	+	Motion artefacts, focus
LSCI	Wide-field ROI: ø 1 cm	-	Non-contact	+	OR lights off
FA	Wide-field ROI: ø 1 cm	-	Non-contact	+	Invasive (ICG injection), OR lights off *

FA Fluorescence Angiography, ICG Indocyanine Green, LSCI Laser Speckle Contrast Imaging, OCT Optical Coherence Tomography, OR Operating Room, ROI Region-of-interest, SDF Sidestream Darkfield Microscopy. * Not when used laparoscopically

3.2. Quantitative Parameters

Of 22 patients, quantitative assessment was successful in 15, 22, 20, and 20 patients for OCT, SDF, LSCI, and FA, respectively. At the four locations (Loc1/Loc2/Loc3/Loc4), the number of obtained measurements for OCT were 12/10/8/10, for SDF 21/21/21/21, for LSCI 20/20/20/20, and for FA 17/20/20/18, respectively. The measurements for the SDF parameters were available in 21 patients at Loc4, except for MFI ($n = 14$).

Comparing Loc1 with Loc4, a significant difference was noticed for 10 out of 14 parameters (Figure 2): the SDF parameters PVD, MFI, PPV, and velocity; the LSCI parameters Flux and Δ%Flux; and the FA parameters influx time point, F_{max}, $T_{1/2}$, and mean slope. Of those, PVD, MFI, PPV, velocity, Flux, F_{max}, and mean slope decreased towards the fundus, while the Δ%Flux, influx time point, and $T_{1/2}$ increased. No significant differences were noticed between the locations for the OCT parameter speckle %, the SDF parameters TVD and DBS, and the FA parameter T_{max}.

Anastomotic leakage occurred in 4/22 patients (18.2%). Of the measurements available at Loc3, anastomotic leakage occurred in 1/8 (12.5%), 3/21 (14.3%), 4/20 (20.0%), and 2/20 (10.0%) for OCT, SDF, LSCI, and FA, respectively. No significant differences were observed for the quantitative parameters between the patients with or without anastomotic leakage at Loc3 (data not shown). Of the measurements available at Loc4, anastomotic leakage occurred in 1/10 (10.0%), 3/21 (14.3%), 4/20 (20.0%), and 2/18 (11.1%) for OCT, SDF, LSCI, and FA, respectively. A comparison of quantitative parameters at Loc4 between patients with and without anastomotic leakage is shown in Table 3. Of all the quantitative parameters, the FA values for the $T_{1/2}$ and mean slope significantly differed between patients with and without anastomotic leakage. The $T_{1/2}$ was 13.0 (total range 6.3–21.3) seconds in patients without anastomotic leakage, and increased to 29.3 (total range 27.8–30.8) seconds in the case of anastomotic leakage ($p = 0.025$). For $T_{1/2}$, the total range of values showed no overlap between patients with or without anastomotic leakage. The mean slope decreased from 1.3 (total range 0.1–11.0) to 0.2 (total range 0.1–0.2) in patients without and with anastomotic leakage ($p = 0.041$), respectively. All the values for the SDF parameters and for Flux were non-significantly higher (Table 3).

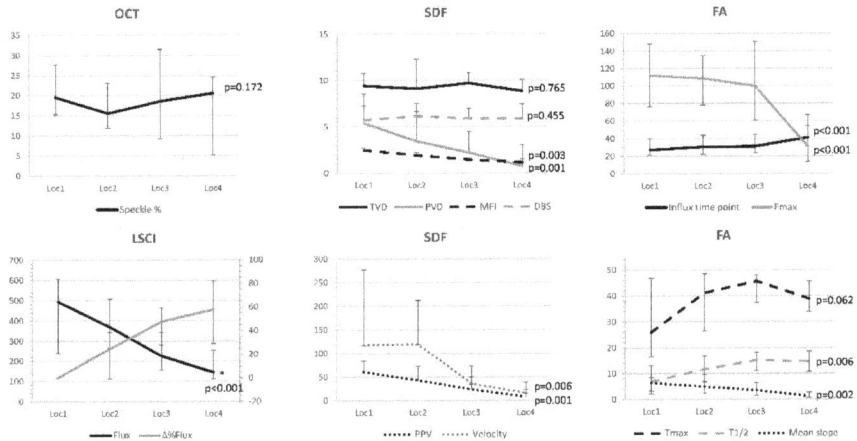

Figure 2. Fourteen quantitative parameters at four locations of the gastric conduit. Data are shown as medians and interquartile ranges. p-value is shown for the difference between Loc1 and Loc4. OCT Optical Coherence Tomography: Speckle in %. SDF Sidestream Darkfield Imaging: TVD total vessel density in mm/mm^2, PVD perfused vessel density in mm/mm^2, MFI microvascular flow index, DBS de Backer score, PPV proportion (%) of perfused vessels. LSCI Laser Speckle Contrast Imaging: Flux in LSPU (laser speckle perfusion units), Δ%Flux percentage difference in Flux relative to Location 1 (right vertical axis). * Not calculated, p-value calculated on absolute data (see Flux). FA Fluorescence Angiography: Influx time point in sec, F_{max} in arbitrary units, T_{max} in sec, $T_{1/2}$ in sec, mean slope in arbitrary units per sec.

Table 3. Comparison of the perfusion-related parameters at location 4 between patients with and without anastomotic leakage.

		Location 4 No Anastomotic Leakage ($n = 18$)	Location 4 Anastomotic Leakage ($n = 4$)	p-Value
OCT	Speckle (%)	21 (14–31)	17 (17)	0.600
SDF	TVD (mm/mm^2)	8.7 (5.1–15.9)	9.8 (9.5–17.4)	0.088
	PVD (mm/mm^2)	0.5 (0.0–7.0)	2.0 (0.9–5.4)	0.155
	MFI	1.1 (0.3–2.0)	1.3 (1–1.5)	0.646
	DBS	5.4 (3.0–10.3)	7.2 (6.9–11.00)	0.056
	PPV (%)	5.7 (0.0–86.4)	21.3 (9.3–31.1)	0.155
	Velocity (μm/s)	15.2 (4.3–186.0)	23.8 (14.8–60.3)	0.560
LSCI	Flux (LSPU)	128.7 (41.1–480.5)	167.1 (114.1–335.2)	0.422
	Δ%Flux (%)	54 (−31–87)	82 (52–87)	0.072
FA	Influx time point (s)	39.5 (21–73)	44.0 (42–46)	0.673
	F_{max} (AU)	39.8 (1.8–163.2)	12.3 (10.9–13.7)	0.131
	T_{max} (s)	38.8 (34.2–44.6)	39.8 (31.1–48.58)	0.888
	$T_{1/2}$ (s)	13.0 (6.3–21.3)	29.3 (27.8–30.8)	*0.025*
	Mean slope (AU/s)	1.3 (0.1–11.0)	0.2 (0.1–0.2)	*0.041*

Data are shown as median and total range. OCT Optical Coherence Tomography, SDF Sidestream Darkfield Imaging, TVD total vessel density in mm/mm^2, PVD perfused vessel density in mm/mm^2, MFI microvascular flow index, DBS de Backer score, PPV proportion (%) of perfused vessels, LSCI Laser Speckle Contrast Imaging, Flux in LSPU (laser speckle perfusion units), Δ%Flux percentage difference in Flux relative to Location 1, FA Fluorescence Angiography, F_{max} in arbitrary units, mean slope in arbitrary units per sec.

At Loc1, the heart rate was correlated with the OCT parameter speckle % ($\rho = 0.669$, $p = 0.017$). Systolic blood pressure was inversely correlated with LSCI parameter Flux ($\rho = -0.451$, $p = 0.046$), and stroke volume with SDF parameter MFI ($\rho = -0.528$, $p = 0.017$). No other significant correlations were observed for the quantitative and hemodynamic parameters.

4. Discussion

Four optical techniques were tested intraoperatively for a quantitative perfusion assessment of the gastric conduit in oesophageal cancer patients undergoing resection. The perfusion restriction towards the fundus was quantitatively assessed and was significantly objectified in 10 out of 14 parameters. At the fundus of the gastric conduit (Loc4), the FA parameters $T_{1/2}$ and mean slope significantly differed between the patients with or without anastomotic leakage.

The gastric conduit is mainly vascularised by the right gastroepiploic artery, which usually terminates before the future anastomotic site, making the future anastomotic site prone to vascularisation problems. Therefore, the gastric conduit is an adequate model for perfusion, as perfusion restriction is expected towards the gastric fundus. Quantitative data from this study indeed showed perfusion restriction towards the fundus. Ten quantitative parameters significantly differed between Loc1 and Loc4, of which seven decreased towards the fundus. Comparing those to the literature, the Flux and F_{max} are described to indicate perfusion restriction towards the fundus [19,20]. Three parameters (Δ%Flux, influx time point (τ), and $T_{1/2}$) increased towards the fundus, indicating decreased perfusion as well. Influx time point (τ) and $T_{1/2}$ measured the time-dependent change in fluorescence. In the literature, the time-dependent change in fluorescence intensity is a potential method for FA quantification, and increased τ and $T_{1/2}$ might indicate inadequate perfusion [19,21–23]. An increase in these values might be due to either diffusion through tissue instead of an intact arterial route or to resistance in the vascular network in the case of venous outflow obstruction.

Quantitative parameters were compared between patients with and without anastomotic leakage at Loc4. In patients with anastomotic leakage, a significantly higher $T_{1/2}$ and significantly lower mean slope were found. $T_{1/2}$ and mean slope provide information about the ICG influx velocity, amount of vessel density, and potentially the outflow. $T_{1/2}$ and mean slope are potentially hands-on parameters for intraoperative perfusion evaluation and anastomotic leakage prediction [19]. At Loc4, in contrast to an expected decrease, the SDF parameters and Flux appeared to be higher for patients with anastomotic leakage compared with patients without leakage. This increase might be explained by venous outflow obstruction. SDF measures the velocity of RBCs using a space–time diagram. The Flux measured by LSCI is dependent on the amount of blood particles and movement of these particles. In the case of venous outflow obstruction at the fundus of the gastric tube, veins swell to 5–10 times their original size [24,25]. The SDF parameters and Flux are possibly influenced by the number of RBCs or blood particles in swollen veins and therefore could be higher at Loc4 in the case of anastomotic leakage secondary to venous outflow obstruction. No differences were observed at Loc4 for the OCT parameter speckle %.

This explorative study allowed the comparison of four optical techniques in terms of their quantitative assessment and imaging characteristics. Both OCT and SDF have a limited field of view focusing on microperfusion, while LSCI and FA are wide-field (considering the heterogeneity of the capillary network). Wide-field techniques allow the immediate overview of entire gastric conduit, and potentially show vascular confines visually, which is valuable for clinical determination of the anastomotic site. Besides, the time consumption for imaging seemed lower for wide-field techniques. OCT, LSCI, and FA are all non-contact techniques, thereby avoiding stabilising problems. Only OCT is depth-resolving (depicting individual overlying vessels). In terms of quantification, quantitative SDF, LCSI, and FA had acceptable success rates. The quantitative parameter for OCT did not significantly differ between Loc1 and Loc4, nor in the case of anastomotic leakage. This observation might be explained by the method of analysis that assessed only one transection of 2.5 mm depth for quantification, indicating that limited field of view techniques might be prone to sampling errors. SDF and LSCI show perfusion restriction towards the fundus, but both show non-significant higher values at Loc4 in the case of anastomotic leakage. As mentioned above, the SDF and LSCI trends might be comparable due to focus on the same perfusion units and might be higher in the case of anastomotic leakage due to venous outflow obstruction. FA visualises the spatial distribution of ICG that is bound to plasma proteins, and thus assesses the patency of vessels and shows vascular confines. FA parameters were able to indicate perfusion restriction towards the fundus as well as in patients with anastomotic leakage. In the case of venous congestion, FA parameters might show resistance in the vasculature, which leads to prolonged time values and a reduced rate in the increase in fluorescence intensity. Furthermore, FA time values might show what degree of arterial diffusion (instead of direct arterial flow) or venous outflow obstruction might lead to anastomotic leakage. Although FA use is dependent on ICG injection, ICG is a safe dye and can be applied at low dosages. Moreover, FA imaging systems are available for laparoscopy, which is clinically beneficial. Therefore, and on the basis of this study, FA quantitative parameters are most promising for future research.

$T_{1/2}$ and mean slope will be promising quantitative parameters for intraoperative clinical decision-making if a threshold can be derived for patient outcomes, including anastomotic leakage. According to the threshold, change in management can include the administration of medication, to shorten the gastric conduit at the maximum extent, or no anastomotic reconstruction and oesophagostomy. The latter option is a very radical solution with a decreased quality of life and need for surgery in the future to make a new reconstruction. Most surgeons would probably choose to make an extra effort to shorten the gastric conduit and make an anastomosis at increased risk instead of choosing no reconstruction as an option. Furthermore, the threshold can be used to identify high-risk patients for anastomotic leakage.

The quantitative parameters for FA may be biased by the duration of imaging, as this might not have been long enough to reach the peak value (F_{max}). This study was further limited by a relatively small number of patients with a low absolute number of anastomotic leakages, and particularly measurements at Loc4 were infrequent. However, this pilot study can guide future studies, by for example serving as a base for sample size calculations. Furthermore, the exact anastomotic site was not recorded, but the anastomosis was constructed between Loc3 and Loc4. At Loc3, no differences were observed for any quantitative parameter, however at Loc4 differences were found. The site of anastomotic reconstruction may have led to bias in the observations. In addition, the system used for SDF measurements involves an older model and older software, and possibly new models (e.g., Cytocam) allow higher resolution, and new software (AVA 5, MicroVision Medical, Amsterdam, The Netherlands) might perform better. However, the SDF technique is still employed, and sampling error and increased values in the case of anastomotic leakage can still be expected. In addition, the parameters were not assessed in relation to patient risk factors. Co-morbidities such as diabetes mellitus and cardiovascular disease affect the (micro) circulation [26,27], and might therefore influence the read-out of the parameters. Furthermore, diabetes mellitus and chronic obstructive pulmonary disease are known risk factors for anastomotic leakage [28]. Owing to the small sample size, correction for co-morbidities was not performed. Nevertheless, it is difficult to compare different optical imaging systems in the literature, and this study allows comparison for the same group of patients. Furthermore, this study evaluated quantitative parameters for both perfusion and patient outcomes.

In conclusion, for future studies, FA and software-derived fluorescence–time curves are most promising to quantitatively assess decreased perfusion (A) towards the fundus in the gastric conduit and (B) in patients with anastomotic leakage. Future FA ideally has a real-time perfusion map with analysis per pixel showing perfusion thresholds. In future studies, FA data should be combined with risk factors for patient outcomes to provide additional information on FA thresholds.

Author Contributions: Conceptualization, M.D.S., S.M.A.J., P.R.B., T.G.v.L., M.I.v.B.H., D.M.d.B., and S.S.G.; Data curation, S.M.A.J.; Formal analysis, M.D.S., S.M.A.J., P.R.B., R.M.v.d.E., and L.S.W.; Investigation, M.I.v.B.H. and S.S.G.; Methodology, S.M.A.J., L.S.W., T.G.v.L., M.I.v.B.H., D.M.d.B. and S.S.G.; Software, P.R.B. and R.M.v.d.E.; Supervision, M.I.v.B.H., D.M.d.B., and S.S.G.; Writing—original draft, M.D.S.; Writing—review and editing, S.M.A.J., P.R.B., R.M.v.d.E., L.S.W., T.G.v.L., M.I.v.B.H., D.M.d.B., and S.S.G. All authors have read and agreed to the published version of the manuscript.

Funding: This research received no external funding.

Conflicts of Interest: M.I.v.B.H.: unrestricted grant and materials Stryker European Operations B.V.; unrestricted grant Olympus; consultant for Medtronic, Johnson & Johnson and Mylan. The other authors declare no conflict of interest.

References

1. Van Hagen, P.; Hulshof, M.C.; van Lanschot, J.J.; Steyerberg, E.W.; van Berge Henegouwen, M.I.; Wijnhoven, B.P.; Richel, D.J.; Nieuwenhuijzen, G.A.; Hospers, G.A.; Bonenkamp, J.J.; et al. Preoperative chemoradiotherapy for esophageal or junctional cancer. *N. Engl. J. Med.* **2012**, *366*, 2074–2084. [CrossRef] [PubMed]
2. Fransen, L.F.C.; Berkelmans, G.H.K.; Asti, E.; van Berge Henegouwen, M.I.; Berlth, F.; Bonavina, L.; Brown, A.; Bruns, C.; van Daele, E.; Gisbertz, S.S.; et al. The Effect of Postoperative Complications After Minimally Invasive Esophagectomy on Long-term Survival: An International Multicenter Cohort Study. *Ann. Surg.* **2020**. [CrossRef] [PubMed]
3. Findlay, J.M.; Gillies, R.S.; Millo, J.; Sgromo, B.; Marshall, R.E.; Maynard, N.D. Enhanced recovery for esophagectomy: A systematic review and evidence-based guidelines. *Ann. Surg.* **2014**, *259*, 413–431. [CrossRef]
4. Fischer, C.; Lingsma, H.; Klazinga, N.; Hardwick, R.; Cromwell, D.; Steyerberg, E.; Groene, O. Volume-outcome revisited: The effect of hospital and surgeon volumes on multiple outcome measures in oesophago-gastric cancer surgery. *PLoS ONE* **2017**, *12*, E0183955. [CrossRef] [PubMed]
5. Jansen, S.M.; de Bruin, D.M.; van Berge Henegouwen, M.I.; Strackee, S.D.; Veelo, D.P.; van Leeuwen, T.G.; Gisbertz, S.S. Optical techniques for perfusion monitoring of the gastric tube after esophagectomy: A review of technologies and thresholds. *Dis. Esophagus Off. J. Int. Soc. Dis. Esophagus* **2018**, *31*. [CrossRef]
6. Van Manen, L.; Handgraaf, H.J.M.; Diana, M.; Dijkstra, J.; Ishizawa, T.; Vahrmeijer, A.L.; Mieog, J.S.D. A practical guide for the use of indocyanine green and methylene blue in fluorescence-guided abdominal surgery. *J. Surg. Oncol.* **2018**, *118*, 283–300. [CrossRef]
7. Jansen, S.M.; de Bruin, D.M.; Faber, D.J.; Dobbe, I.; Heeg, E.; Milstein, D.M.J.; Strackee, S.D.; van Leeuwen, T.G. Applicability of quantitative optical imaging techniques for intraoperative perfusion diagnostics: A comparison of laser speckle contrast imaging, sidestream dark-field microscopy, and optical coherence tomography. *J. Biomed. Opt.* **2017**, *22*, 086004. [CrossRef]
8. Prasetya, H.; Jansen, S.M.; Marquering, H.A.; van Leeuwen, T.G.; Gisbertz, S.S.; de Bruin, D.M.; van Bavel, E. Estimation of microvascular perfusion after esophagectomy: A quantitative model of dynamic fluorescence imaging. *Med. Biol. Eng. Comput.* **2019**, *57*, 1889–1990. [CrossRef]
9. AV, D.S.; Lin, H.; Henderson, E.R.; Samkoe, K.S.; Pogue, B.W. Review of fluorescence guided surgery systems: Identification of key performance capabilities beyond indocyanine green imaging. *J. Biomed. Opt.* **2016**, *21*, 80901. [CrossRef]
10. Bossuyt, P.M.; Reitsma, J.B.; Bruns, D.E.; Gatsonis, C.A.; Glasziou, P.P.; Irwig, L.M.; Moher, D.; Rennie, D.; de Vet, H.C.; Lijmer, J.G. The STARD statement for reporting studies of diagnostic accuracy: Explanation and elaboration. *Clin. Chem.* **2003**, *49*, 7–18. [CrossRef]
11. Vandenbroucke, J.P.; von Elm, E.; Altman, D.G.; Gotzsche, P.C.; Mulrow, C.D.; Pocock, S.J.; Poole, C.; Schlesselman, J.J.; Egger, M. Strengthening the Reporting of Observational Studies in Epidemiology (STROBE): Explanation and elaboration. *Int. J. Surg. (Lond. Engl.)* **2014**, *12*, 1500–1524. [CrossRef] [PubMed]
12. Jansen, S.M.; de Bruin, D.M.; van Berge Henegouwen, M.I.; Strackee, S.D.; Veelo, D.P.; van Leeuwen, T.G.; Gisbertz, S.S. Can we predict necrosis intra-operatively? Real-time optical quantitative perfusion imaging in surgery: Study protocol for a prospective, observational, in vivo pilot study. *Pilot Feasibility Stud.* **2017**, *3*, 65. [CrossRef] [PubMed]
13. Hagens, E.R.C.; Künzli, H.T.; van Rijswijk, A.S.; Meijer, S.L.; Mijnals, R.C.D.; Weusten, B.; Geijsen, E.D.; van Laarhoven, H.W.M.; van Berge Henegouwen, M.I.; Gisbertz, S.S. Distribution of lymph node metastases in esophageal adenocarcinoma after neoadjuvant chemoradiation therapy: A prospective study. *Surg. Endosc.* **2019**. [CrossRef]
14. Jansen, S.M.; Almasian, M.; Wilk, L.S.; de Bruin, D.M.; van Berge Henegouwen, M.I.; Strackee, S.D.; Bloemen, P.R.; Meijer, S.L.; Gisbertz, S.S.; van Leeuwen, T.G. Feasibility of Optical Coherence Tomography (OCT) for Intra-Operative Detection of Blood Flow during Gastric Tube Reconstruction. *Sensors* **2018**, *18*, 1331. [CrossRef] [PubMed]

15. De Backer, D.; Hollenberg, S.; Boerma, C.; Goedhart, P.; Büchele, G.; Ospina-Tascon, G.; Dobbe, I.; Ince, C. How to evaluate the microcirculation: Report of a round table conference. *Crit. Care (Lond. Engl.)* **2007**, *11*, R101. [CrossRef] [PubMed]
16. Balestra, G.M.; Bezemer, R.; Boerma, E.C.; Yong, Z.Y.; Sjauw, K.D.; Engstrom, A.E.; Koopmans, M.; Ince, C. Improvement of sidestream dark field imaging with an image acquisition stabilizer. *BMC Med. Imaging* **2010**, *10*, 15. [CrossRef]
17. Jansen, S.M.; de Bruin, D.M.; van Berge Henegouwen, M.I.; Bloemen, P.R.; Strackee, S.D.; Veelo, D.P.; van Leeuwen, T.G.; Gisbertz, S.S. Effect of ephedrine on gastric conduit perfusion measured by laser speckle contrast imaging after esophagectomy: A prospective in vivo cohort study. *Dis. Esophagus Off. J. Int. Soc. Dis. Esophagus* **2018**, *31*, doy031. [CrossRef]
18. Low, D.E.; Alderson, D.; Cecconello, I.; Chang, A.C.; Darling, G.E.; D'Journo, X.B.; Griffin, S.M.; Holscher, A.H.; Hofstetter, W.L.; Jobe, B.A.; et al. International Consensus on Standardization of Data Collection for Complications Associated With Esophagectomy: Esophagectomy Complications Consensus Group (ECCG). *Ann. Surg.* **2015**, *262*, 286–294. [CrossRef]
19. Slooter, M.D.; Mansvelders, M.S.E.; Bloemen, P.R.; Gisbertz, S.S.; Bemelman, W.A.; Tanis, P.J.; Hompes, R.; van Berge Henegouwen, M.I.; de Bruin, D.M. Defining indocyanine green fluorescence to assess anastomotic perfusion during gastrointestinal surgery: Systematic review. *BJS Open* **2020**, in press.
20. Milstein, D.M.; Ince, C.; Gisbertz, S.S.; Boateng, K.B.; Geerts, B.F.; Hollmann, M.W.; van Berge Henegouwen, M.I.; Veelo, D.P. Laser speckle contrast imaging identifies ischemic areas on gastric tube reconstructions following esophagectomy. *Medicine* **2016**, *95*, e3875. [CrossRef]
21. Kamiya, K.; Unno, N.; Miyazaki, S.; Sano, M.; Kikuchi, H.; Hiramatsu, Y.; Ohta, M.; Yamatodani, T.; Mineta, H.; Konno, H. Quantitative assessment of the free jejunal graft perfusion. *J. Surg. Res.* **2015**, *194*, 394–399. [CrossRef]
22. Kumagai, Y.; Hatano, S.; Sobajima, J.; Ishiguro, T.; Fukuchi, M.; Ishibashi, K.I.; Mochiki, E.; Nakajima, Y.; Ishida, H. Indocyanine green fluorescence angiography of the reconstructed gastric tube during esophagectomy: Efficacy of the 90-second rule. *Dis. Esophagus Off. J. Int. Soc. Dis. Esophagus* **2018**, *31*. [CrossRef]
23. Koyanagi, K.; Ozawa, S.; Oguma, J.; Kazuno, A.; Yamazaki, Y.; Ninomiya, Y.; Ochiai, H.; Tachimori, Y. Blood flow speed of the gastric conduit assessed by indocyanine green fluorescence: New predictive evaluation of anastomotic leakage after esophagectomy. *Medicine* **2016**, *95*, e4386. [CrossRef] [PubMed]
24. Murakami, M.; Sugiyama, A.; Ikegami, T.; Ishida, K.; Maruta, F.; Shimizu, F.; Ikeno, T.; Kawasaki, S. Revascularization using the short gastric vessels of the gastric tube after subtotal esophagectomy for intrathoracic esophageal carcinoma. *J. Am. Coll. Surg.* **2000**, *190*, 71–77. [CrossRef]
25. Buise, M.P.; Ince, C.; Tilanus, H.W.; Klein, J.; Gommers, D.; van Bommel, J. The effect of nitroglycerin on microvascular perfusion and oxygenation during gastric tube reconstruction. *Anesth. Analg.* **2005**, *100*, 1107–1111. [CrossRef] [PubMed]
26. Mcmillan, D.E. Development of vascular complications in diabetes. *Vasc. Med.* **1997**, *2*, 132–142. [CrossRef] [PubMed]
27. Strain, W.D.; Paldánius, P.M. Diabetes, cardiovascular disease and the microcirculation. *Cardiovasc. Diabetol.* **2018**, *17*, 57. [CrossRef] [PubMed]
28. Gooszen, J.A.H.; Goense, L.; Gisbertz, S.S.; Ruurda, J.P.; van Hillegersberg, R.; van Berge Henegouwen, M.I. Intrathoracic versus cervical anastomosis and predictors of anastomotic leakage after oesophagectomy for cancer. *Br. J. Surg.* **2018**, *105*, 552–560. [CrossRef]

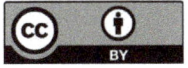

© 2020 by the authors. Licensee MDPI, Basel, Switzerland. This article is an open access article distributed under the terms and conditions of the Creative Commons Attribution (CC BY) license (http://creativecommons.org/licenses/by/4.0/).

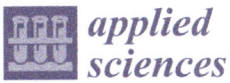

Article

Optimal Spectral Combination of a Hyperspectral Camera for Intraoperative Hemodynamic and Metabolic Brain Mapping

Charly Caredda [1],*, Laurent Mahieu-Williame [1], Raphaël Sablong [1], Michaël Sdika [1], Jacques Guyotat [2] and Bruno Montcel [1],*

[1] Université de Lyon, INSA-Lyon, Université Claude Bernard Lyon 1, UJM-Saint Etienne, CNRS, Inserm, CREATIS UMR 5220, U1206, F69100 Lyon, France; Laurent.Mahieu-Williame@creatis.insa-lyon.fr (L.M.-W.); Raphael.Sablong@creatis.insa-lyon.fr (R.S.); Michael.Sdika@creatis.insa-lyon.fr (M.S.)

[2] Service de Neurochirurgie D, Hospices Civils de Lyon, F69500 Bron, France; jacques.guyotat@chu-lyon.fr

* Correspondence: charly.caredda@creatis.insa-lyon.fr (C.C.); bruno.montcel@univ-lyon1.fr (B.M.)

Received: 24 June 2020; Accepted: 21 July 2020 ; Published: 27 July 2020

Abstract: Intraoperative optical imaging is a localization technique for the functional areas of the human brain cortex during neurosurgical procedures. These areas are assessed by monitoring the oxygenated (HbO_2) and deoxygenated hemoglobin (Hb) concentration changes occurring in the brain. Sometimes, the functional status of the brain is assessed using metabolic biomarkers: the oxidative state of cytochrome-c-oxidase (oxCCO). A setup composed of a white light source and a hyperspectral or a standard RGB camera could be used to identify the functional areas. The choice of the best spectral configuration is still based on an empirical approach. We propose in this study a method to define the optimal spectral combinations of a commercial hyperspectral camera for the computation of hemodynamic and metabolic brain maps. The method is based on a Monte Carlo framework that simulates the acquisition of the intrinsic optical signal following a neuronal activation. The results indicate that the optimal spectral combination of a hyperspectral camera aims to accurately quantify the HbO_2 (0.5% error), Hb (4.4% error), and oxCCO (15% error) responses in the brain following neuronal activation. We also show that RGB imaging is a low cost and accurate solution to compute Hb maps (4% error), but not accurate to compute HbO_2 (48% error) or oxCCO (1036% error) maps.

Keywords: hemodynamic brain mapping; metabolic brain mapping; Monte Carlo simulations; intraoperative imaging; optical imaging; hyperspectral imaging; RGB imaging

1. Introduction

Non-invasive functional brain mapping is an imaging technique used to localize the functional areas of the patient brain. This technique is used during brain tumor resection surgery to indicate to the neurosurgeon the cortical tissues that should not be removed without cognitive impairment. Functional magnetic resonance imaging (fMRI) [1] is the preoperative gold standard for the identification of the patient brain functional areas. However, after patient craniotomy, a brain shift invalidates the relevance of neuro-navigation to intraoperatively localize the functional areas of the patient brain [2]. In order to prevent any localization error, intraoperative MRI has been suggested, but it complicates the surgery gesture, which makes it rarely used. For these reasons, electrical brain stimulation [3] is preferred during neurosurgery. However, this technique suffers from limitations because the measurements could trigger epilepsy seizures. Since optical imaging combined with a quantitative modeling of brain hemodynamic biomarkers could evaluate in real time the functional areas during neurosurgery [4–6], this technique could serve as a tool of choice to complement the electrical brain stimulation.

Hyperspectral imaging allows the in vivo monitoring of the hemodynamic and metabolic status of an exposed cortex. Hyperspectral imaging provides spatially and spectrally resolved images using numerous and contiguous spectral bands [7]. In comparison, a standard color camera (or RGB camera) acquires three colors (red, green, and blue) using broad and overlapping spectral detectors. Both techniques have the ability to measure the oxygenation changes in the tissue using the modified Beer–Lambert law [5,8–12]. In functional brain mapping studies, the concentration changes of oxy- (ΔC_{HbO_2}) and deoxy-hemoglobin (ΔC_{Hb}) can be analyzed to identify the activated cortical areas [5,13–21]. The acquisition of the intrinsic signal in the near-infrared range offers the potential to monitor the brain metabolism with the quantification of the concentration changes of the oxidative state of cytochrome-c-oxidase (ΔC_{oxCCO}) [22–25]. Hyperspectral and color cameras combined with a white light illumination are simple and powerful tools for the computation of intraoperative functional brain maps. The objective is to guide the neurosurgeon during brain surgery to prevent any functional impairments after surgical procedures (tumor resection).

In the literature, all wavelength bands acquired by hyperspectral imaging setups are used to measure the hemodynamic and metabolic changes in the brain [10,24–26]. However, there are some studies in which the choice of the selected spectral bands is discussed. Bale et al. [23] showed that tens to hundreds of spectral bands acquired with a broadband near-infrared spectroscopy setup (780 nm to 900 nm) can be used to measure the oxCCO concentration changes. Arifler et al. [27] showed that eight wavelength combinations between 780 nm and 900 nm give rise to the least possible estimation errors for the deconvolution of ΔC_{HbO_2}, ΔC_{Hb}, and ΔC_{oxCCO} when compared to a gold standard (121 wavelengths included between 780 nm and 900 nm). Giannoni et al. [28] proposed a Monte Carlo framework to investigate the performances of broadband spectroscopy to quantify the brain hemodynamic and metabolic responses. The results of this study indicated that eight wavelength between 780 nm and 900 nm should be selected to provide minimal differences in quantification compared to a gold standard of 121 wavelengths (780 nm to 900 nm). Sudakou et al. [29] proposed a method based on the error propagation analysis and Monte Carlo simulations (three layer model: scalp, skull, and brain) allowing the estimation of the cytochrome-c-oxidase uncertainty in data measured with a multispectral time-resolved near-infrared spectroscopy device. The results of this study indicated that 16 wavelengths between 688 and 875 nm could be used to minimize the standard deviation of the cytochrome-c-oxidase concentration changes in the brain layer. Wavelength optimization problems have also been studied for other optical imaging techniques such as near-infrared optical tomography. Chen et al. [30] identified seven laser diodes among 38 commercially available diodes in the range of 633–980 nm to estimate four chromophores (HbO_2, Hb, water, and lipids) and the scattering prefactor in breast tissue. Chen et al. used the condition number and the residual norm to identify the optimal matrix used for the resolution of a linear system and thus to estimate four chromophores and the scattering prefactor in breast tissue. The optimal wavelengths were identified for a large residual norm and small condition number. The residual norm and the condition number can be interpreted as parameters representing the uniqueness and stability of the solution, respectively.

The commercial hyperspectral cameras have limited choices in the available spectral bands and do not have a spectral resolution as high as the broadband spectroscopy devices used by Bale et al. and Arifler et al. Therefore, the optimal spectral bands identified in these studies may not be available with the commercial cameras. Moreover, the more spectral bands are used, the more time is needed to compute functional brain maps. Since time is the key factor in intraoperative imaging, the smallest number of spectral bands must be acquired while ensuring minimal quantification errors.

First, we propose in this study a method to define the optimal spectral combinations of a commercial hyperspectral camera for intraoperative hemodynamic and metabolic brain mapping. This method could be used with any hyperspectral or standard RGB camera to evaluate its ability to compute accurate hemodynamic (ΔC_{HbO_2} and ΔC_{Hb}) and/or metabolic (ΔC_{oxCCO}) brain maps following neuronal activation. The method is based on the Monte Carlo simulations of the acquisition of the intrinsic signal acquired by a camera. All spectral combinations of the hyperspectral camera are tested to evaluate the optimal spectral configuration that minimize the quantification errors in

ΔC_{HbO_2}, ΔC_{Hb}, and ΔC_{oxCCO}. In this work, we also show that a spectral correction [10] of the reflection spectra acquired by a mosaic hyperspectral sensor is mandatory to minimize the chromophores' quantification errors. Finally, we compare standard RGB imaging and hyperspectral imaging for hemodynamic and metabolic brain mapping. We demonstrate that RGB imaging is a low cost, but not an accurate solution to identify the functional areas in a patient brain based on the analysis of the cortical hemodynamics. Hyperspectral imaging is the ideal solution for an accurate computation of hemodynamic and metabolic brain maps.

2. Materials and Methods

We simulated the acquisition of the intrinsic reflection spectra of a patient exposed cortex using hyperspectral imaging to determine the optimal spectral configuration for the computation of hemodynamic and/or metabolic brain maps. We also simulated the acquisition of the intrinsic reflection spectra based on standard RGB imaging to evaluate the potential benefit of using hyperspectral imaging.

2.1. Simulated Setup

In this study, the imaging system represented in Figure 1 was simulated. This setup was used in our previous study [5] for the identification of functional areas based on RGB imaging. A continuous wave white light source illuminated the patient exposed cortex. The light source was a halogen bulb (OSRAM Classic 116W 230V) whose spectra was measured with a USB 2000 spectrometer [31]. The intrinsic reflection spectra were acquired by a hyperspectral camera (XIMEA MQ022HG-IM-SM5X5-NIR) and standard RGB camera (BASLER acA2000-165uc). Both RGB and hyperspectral cameras acquire spectrally and spatially resolved images, but these two systems differ in their spectral resolution. The RGB camera acquires three broad and overlapping spectra over 300 nm to 700 nm using a Bayer filter [32] mounted on a CMOS sensor. The hyperspectral camera acquires 25 narrow and contiguous spectral bands in the red in the near-infrared range. A 5 × 5 mosaic filter (25 Fabry–Perot filters) mounted on a CMOS sensor was used for the acquisition of the 25 spectral bands. Each Fabry–Perot filter has two transmission peaks. The first or the second peak can be selected by mounting an interference filter on the camera lens. In our study, a long pass filter mounted on the hyperspectral camera lens selected the wavelength included between 675 nm and 975 nm.

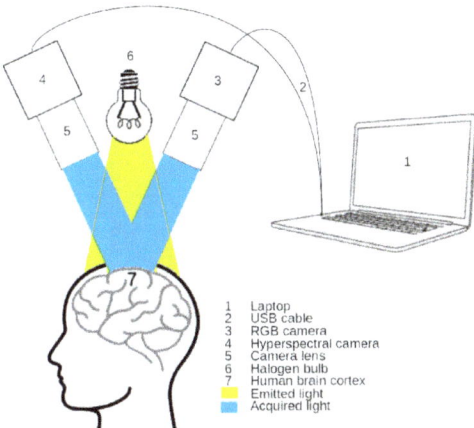

Figure 1. Schematic of the simulated imaging system.

The intensity R measured by the spectral channel k of the camera ($k \in [1;3]$ for RGB imaging and $k \in [1;25]$ for hyperspectral imaging) is expressed by the following equation:

$$R_k = \int_{\lambda_{min}}^{\lambda_{max}} D_k(\lambda).\Phi(\lambda).d\lambda. \tag{1}$$

The integral runs from $\lambda_{min} = 400$ nm to $\lambda_{max} = 700$ nm for RGB imaging and from $\lambda_{min} = 675$ nm to $\lambda_{max} = 975$ nm for hyperspectral imaging. These wavelengths delimit the ranges of the spectral sensitivity profiles provided by the camera manufacturers. D_k is the spectral sensitivity of spectral channel k of the camera, provided by the camera manufacturer. Φ is the diffuse reflection spectra of the illuminated tissue.

2.2. Hyperspectral Correction

In hyperspectral imaging based on mosaic filters, the use of the interference filter does not completely eliminate the crosstalk between the camera spectral sensitivities. To approach the ideal spectral sensitivity D^{ideal} (provided by the camera manufacturer), Pichette et al. [10] proposed to compute a linear combination of the spectral sensitivities:

$$D_m^{Corr}(\lambda) = \sum_{k=1}^{25} X_{m,k}.D_k(\lambda) \tag{2}$$

with D_m^{Corr} the corrected spectral sensibility of the spectral channel m ($m \in [1;25]$) and X the 25×25 correction matrix. This correction matrix X was computed with a linear least squares fitting:

$$\min_X \|D^{ideal} - X.D\|_2^2, \tag{3}$$

The normalized spectral sensitivities ($\int D(\lambda).d\lambda = 1$) are represented in Figure 2.

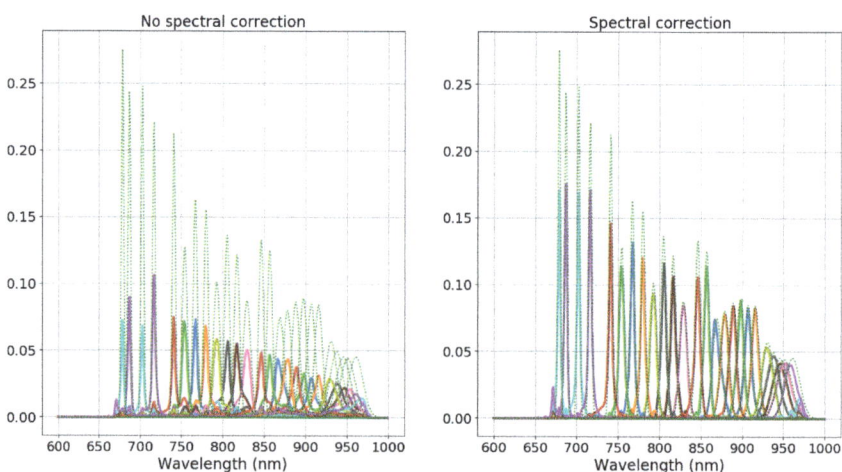

Figure 2. Spectral sensitivities of the hyperspectral camera XIMEA MQ022HG-IM-SM5X5-NIR. The uncorrected spectral sensitivities are plotted in solid lines on the left side of the figure and the corrected ones on the right side. The ideal spectral sensitivities are plotted in green dashed lines.

As the normalized spectral sensitivity ($\int D(\lambda).d\lambda = 1$) represents a probability density function, the Kullback–Leibler divergence can be used to quantify the performance of the spectral correction [33]:

$$KL_k(D_k \| D_k^{ideal}) = \int_{\lambda_{min}}^{\lambda_{max}} D_k(\lambda). \log\left(\frac{D_k(\lambda)}{D_k^{ideal}(\lambda)}\right) d\lambda. \tag{4}$$

$KL_k(D_k \| D_k^{ideal})$ represents the Kullback–Leibler divergence (KL divergence) computed between the spectral sensitivity of the channel k (corrected or uncorrected) and the ideal spectral sensitivity of the channel k. The KL divergence represents a measure of dissimilarity between D_k and D_k^{ideal}. A value equal to 0 indicates the equality of the two probability density functions. The KL divergence values computed for the corrected and uncorrected spectral sensitivities are represented in Figure 3.

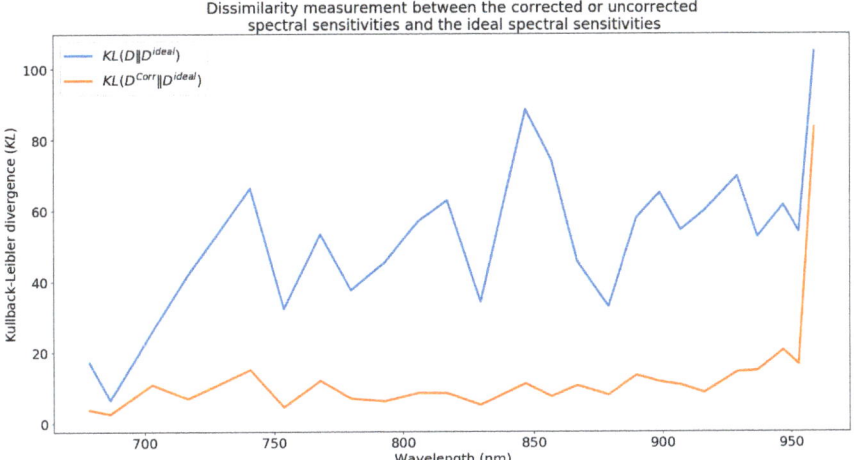

Figure 3. Measure of dissimilarities between the corrected (in orange) or uncorrected (in blue) spectral sensibilities and the ideal spectral sensitivities.

The KL divergence computed between the uncorrected spectral sensitivities and the ideal spectral sensitivities is on average four times higher than those computed between the corrected spectral sensitivities and the ideal spectral sensitivities.

2.3. Sensor Signal-to-Noise Ratio

The signal-to-noise ratios (SNR) of the spectral channel k of the RGB and hyperspectral cameras were measured by acquiring the white light reflected at the surface of a calibration target (plain white sheet of paper) during two minutes with an integration time set to 33 ms:

$$SNR(k) = \frac{\mu_k}{\sigma_k}. \quad (5)$$

μ_k denotes the spectral channel k mean value obtained by computing the mean value of the temporal intensity averaged over the sensor area. σ_k is the spectral channel k standard deviation value obtained by computing the standard deviation value of the temporal intensity averaged over the sensor area. The illumination source power, quantum efficiency and integration time of the cameras directly impact the SNR values. The SNR values of the RGB and hyperspectral cameras we used in this study are represented in Figure 4. The SNR of the red channel of the RGB camera is 1.1 times greater than the one of the green channel and 1.4 times greater than the one of the blue channel. The mean value of the SNR of the hyperspectral is 3.9 times lower than the SNR value of the red channel of the RGB camera. Note that these values are dependent on our experimental configuration and directly impact the amount of noise and the quantification error in the simulated concentration changes.

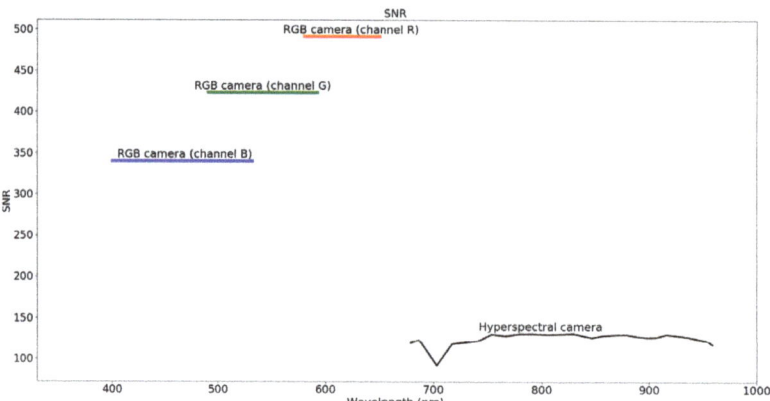

Figure 4. SNR values of each spectral channel of the RGB and hyperspectral cameras.

2.4. Simulation of the Patient Cortical Activation

Following the patient physiological activity, a hemodynamic change occurs in the activated cortical areas with an increase of the oxygenated hemoglobin concentration (C_{HbO_2}) and a decrease of the deoxygenated hemoglobin concentration changes (C_{Hb}). These hemodynamic changes are not the only ones that occur during a patient physiological activity. The concentration of the oxidative state of cytochrome-c-oxidase (C_{oxCCO}) also varies [22]. Cytochrome-c-oxidase (CCO) is an enzyme in the mitochondria that is involved in the aerobic metabolism of glucose. The total concentration of CCO does not change over a short time period (in the order of hours). However, it is possible to assess the differences between the oxidized and reduced states of CCO to obtain an indicator of the change in the CCO redox state.

The patient cortical activation was simulated by Monte Carlo simulations [34]. A volume of 60 mm × 60 mm × 60 mm of grey matter was modeled under a homogeneous white light illumination. Each voxel of the modeled tissue included the information of optical parameters (absorption μ_a, scattering μ_s, anisotropy g coefficients, and refractive index n). A white light illumination was simulated by scanning the optical parameters along the entire illumination spectrum (from 400 nm to 1000 nm in steps of 1 nm). The size of the modeled tissues was chosen in accordance with the photon sensitivity profile [5,35] computed for the detector situated at the center of the top face of the volumes. To avoid any photon loss and inexact results due to the boundary conditions (the simulation of the travel of a packet of photon stops when this packet of photon leaves the volume), the size of the models was set to 60 × 60 × 60 voxels with a resolution of 1 mm^3. The 10^8 packets of photons were homogeneously illuminating the modeled surface. The optical mean path length and the diffuse reflection spectra were measured at the detector position with an integration time set to 33 ms, and the diffuse reflection spectra was normalized to a unitary source.

The optical parameters were taken from the literature and correspond to a nominal physiological condition [36–41]. The anisotropy, reduced scattering coefficients, and the refractive index used in the Monte Carlo simulations are summarized in Table 1. The scattering coefficient μ_s was calculated from the reduced scattering coefficient (μ'_s) and the anisotropy coefficient (g): $\mu_s = \mu'_s/(1-g)$. In Table 1, λ denotes the wavelength dependence of the reduced scattering coefficient (in nm).

Table 1. Anisotropy, reduced scattering coefficients, and refractive index used in the Monte Carlo simulations.

Anisotropy Coefficient g	Reduced Scattering Coefficient μ'_s (cm^{-1})	Refractive Index n
0.85 [42]	$40.8 \cdot \frac{\lambda}{500}^{-3.089}$ [39]	1.36 [38]

The absorption coefficients were calculated using the chemical composition of the chromophores of the simulated tissues, which are summarized in Table 2.

Table 2. Chemical composition of the chromophores of the simulated volumes of grey matter.

	Non-Activated Grey Matter	Activated Grey Matter
Water	73%	73%
C_{Hb} (µmol·L^{-1})	22.1	18.35
C_{HbO_2} (µmol·L^{-1})	65.1	70.1
C_{oxCCO} (µmol·L^{-1})	5.3	5.8

The chemical differences between the activated and non-activated grey matter are represented by a 5 µmol·L^{-1} increase of C_{HbO_2}, a 3.75 µmol·L^{-1} decrease of C_{Hb}, and a 0.5 µmol·L^{-1} increase of C_{oxCCO}. These concentration changes are consistent with those defined in the literature. The reflection spectra and the optical mean path length were measured at the center of the top face of the volume.

2.5. Modified Beer–Lambert Law

The modified Beer–Lambert law is used to convert the acquired intrinsic reflection spectra into concentration changes. Optical functional brain maps are computed by assessing the oxy- and deoxy-genated hemoglobin concentration changes (ΔC_{HbO_2} and ΔC_{Hb}) [9,10,43]. Using the near-infrared range, the oxidative state of cytochrome-c-oxidase concentration changes (ΔC_{oxCCO}) can also be quantified [23]. The modified Beer–Lambert law can be expressed as a linear system [9]:

$$\begin{bmatrix} \Delta A_1 \\ \vdots \\ \Delta A_N \end{bmatrix} = \begin{bmatrix} E_{1,HbO_2} & E_{1,Hb} & E_{1,oxCCO} \\ \vdots & \vdots & \vdots \\ E_{N,HbO_2} & E_{N,Hb} & E_{N,oxCCO} \end{bmatrix} \times \begin{bmatrix} \Delta C_{HbO_2} \\ \Delta C_{Hb} \\ \Delta C_{oxCCO} \end{bmatrix} \quad (6)$$

with

$$E_{k,n} = \int \epsilon_n(\lambda).D_k(\lambda).S(\lambda).L(\lambda).d\lambda. \quad (7)$$

ΔA_k is the absorbance changes measured by the spectral channel k of the camera ($k \in [1;N]$ with $N \in [3;25]$ for hyperspectral imaging and $k \in [1;3]$ for RGB imaging):

$$\Delta A_k = \log_{10}\left(\frac{R_k^{GM_1}}{R_k^{GM_2}}\right). \quad (8)$$

$R_k^{GM_1}$ is the intensity of the non-activated grey matter (see Section 2.4) acquired by the spectral channel k of the camera. $R_k^{GM_2}$ is the intensity of the activated grey matter (see Section 2.4) acquired by the spectral channel k of the camera. The intensities were calculated with Equation (1) using the reflection spectra simulated by Monte Carlo simulations. ΔC_{Hb} is the deoxygenated hemoglobin molar concentration changes (in mol·L^{-1}). ΔC_{HbO_2} is the oxygenated hemoglobin molar concentration changes (in mol·L^{-1}) and ΔC_{oxCCO} the oxidative state of cytochrome-c-oxidase concentration changes (in mol·L^{-1}). ϵ_n is the extinction coefficient of the chromophore n (in L·mol^{-1}·cm^{-1}). The spectral sensitivity of the channel k is represented by $D_k(\lambda)$, and $S(\lambda)$ is the normalized intensity spectrum of the light source. $L(\lambda)$ is the wavelength dependent mean optical path length of the photons traveling in tissue estimated by Monte Carlo simulations (in cm); see Section 2.4. The concentration changes were obtained by matrix inversion once the matrix E was calculated.

2.6. Determination of the Optimal Spectral Configuration of the Hyperspectral Camera

The quantification of ΔC_{Hb}, ΔC_{HbO_2}, and ΔC_{oxCCO} can be achieved using at least three wavelengths [44]. With our hyperspectral camera, twenty-five spectral bands were acquired.

Therefore, we can then ask ourselves what is the optimal spectral configuration for the assessment of ΔC_{Hb}, ΔC_{HbO_2}, and ΔC_{oxCCO}? If N spectral bands were used ($N \in [3;25]$), P combinations may be investigated:

$$\forall N \in [3;25] \quad P = \frac{25!}{(25-N)! \times N!} \tag{9}$$

2.6.1. Noise in Simulations

In order to evaluate the robustness of the chromophores' quantification, zero mean Gaussian noises were added to the simulated quantities. The Monte Carlo noises (noise on diffuse reflection spectra ϕ and mean path length L) were estimated for each simulated wavelength by launching the MCX software 10^3 times using random seeds. The seed is a number used to generate a random number with a pseudorandom number generator. For each wavelength, the standard deviations of the Monte Carlo noises were measured on these 10^3 simulations. The Monte Carlo noise depends on the number of packets of photons used in the simulation. In addition, the noise of the hyperspectral and RGB cameras that were experimentally measured (see Section 2.3) were added to the simulated intensities.

2.6.2. Simulation Based Method

For all the possible P combinations for a group of N spectral bands (see Equation (9)), the quantification errors in ΔC_{Hb}, ΔC_{HbO_2}, or ΔC_{oxCCO} were computed:

$$E_{\Delta C_n}(N, p) = \left| \frac{\Delta C_n^{Expected} - \Delta C_n^{Estimated}(N, p)}{\Delta C_n^{Expected}} \right| \times 100. \tag{10}$$

Note that this quantification error is represented in absolute values. $\Delta C_n^{Expected}$ is the concentration changes of the chromophore n that were expected to be measured in the tissue; see Section 2.4. $\Delta C_n^{Estimated}(N, p)$ is the concentration changes of the chromophore n estimated from the simulated data using the combination p ($p \in [1; P]$) for a group of N spectral bands; see Equation (9). The computation of $\Delta C_n^{Estimated}(N, p)$ and $E_{\Delta C_n}(N, p)$ was repeated 10^3 times to get their mean and the standard deviation values. Different noises were added to the simulated reflection spectra ϕ, mean path length L, and camera intensities R for each iteration. For each group of N spectral bands, the optimal spectral combination among the P possibilities was determined using Equation (11):

$$\min_{p} \left(\sqrt{m\left(E_{\Delta C_n}(N, p)\right)^2 + \sigma\left(E_{\Delta C_n}(N, p)\right)^2} \right). \tag{11}$$

m and σ designate the mean and standard deviation functions, respectively. This metric was chosen to identify the spectral combination of N spectral bands that minimize the average quantification errors while ensuring the reproduction of measurements. Equation (11) leads to the determination of the combination p_n^N, which is the best combination of N spectral bands for the deconvolution of the chromophore n. Finally, the optimal spectral configurations of the hyperspectral camera for the quantification of ΔC_{HbO_2}, ΔC_{Hb}, and ΔC_{oxCCO} were obtained using Equation (12):

$$\min_{p_n^N} \left(\sqrt{m\left(E_{\Delta C_n}(N, p_n^N)\right)^2 + \sigma\left(E_{\Delta C_n}(N, p_n^N)\right)^2} \right). \tag{12}$$

Note that the spectral configurations determined by Equation (12) are not necessarily the same for the deconvolution of ΔC_{HbO_2}, ΔC_{Hb}, and ΔC_{oxCCO}. In other words, this means that three distinct configurations may be used.

2.7. Application to a Functional Brain Mapping Study

In functional brain mapping studies, the measured hemodynamic concentration changes' time courses are compared to the patient theoretical hemodynamic responses. These theoretical responses are obtained by convolving the hemodynamic impulse response function to the window function representing the patient physiological stimulus. The functional areas may be identified by testing the Pearson correlation coefficients (computed between the concentration changes' time courses and the theoretical hemodynamic responses) and the concentration changes averaged over the patient activity period with several T-tests [5,25]. Another technique derived by BOLD fMRI (blood oxygenation level dependent, functional magnetic resonance imaging) is the NIRS SPM (near-infrared spectroscopy statistical parametric mapping) analyses [13,14] that use a general linear model and random field theory to identify the functional areas in a pixel-wise manner.

We built a simulation of the grey matter hemodynamic and metabolic responses following a patient physiological stimulus based on the Monte Carlo framework described in Section 2.4. The intrinsic signal was acquired during 60 s at 0.5 frames per second with the integration time set to 33 ms. The following paradigm was simulated: 18 s of rest, 20 s of neuronal stimulation, followed by 22 s of rest. We incorporated the temporal hemodynamic response, as well as the temporal oxCCO response following neuronal activation. The hemodynamic responses were obtained by convolving the hemodynamic impulse response function to the window function representing the patient physiological stimulus. The oxCCO response function was introduced by Wobst et al. [45] to describe the metabolic response in the primary and adjacent visual cortex for a stimulus of 6 to 24 s. The theoretical time courses can be roughly represented by the function $h(t) = a.t^2.e^{-t}$ convolved with the window function representing the patient physiological stimulus. In this function, t represents the time (in s) and a is the characteristic amplitude of ΔC_{oxCCO}. The theoretical temporal variation of the ΔC_{HbO_2}, ΔC_{Hb}, and ΔC_{oxCCO} values are represented in Figure 5. Note that these values varied homogeneously in the modeled tissue. During these absorption perturbations, the other optical coefficients were kept constant.

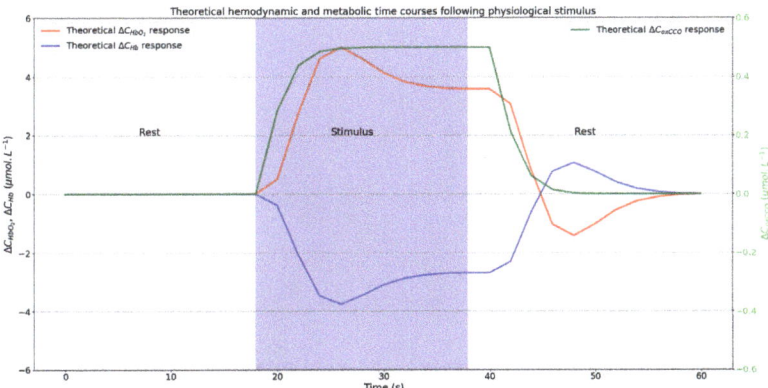

Figure 5. Theoretical ΔC_{HbO_2} (in red), ΔC_{Hb} (in blue), and ΔC_{oxCCO} (in green) responses following the patient physiological activity. ΔC_{HbO_2} and ΔC_{Hb} are expressed by the left vertical axis. ΔC_{oxCCO} is expressed by the right vertical axis. The blue rectangle represent the "patient" physiological stimulus.

With these simulations, we can evaluate the potential benefit from using hyperspectral imaging for the computation of hemodynamic brain maps instead of using a standard RGB camera (see our previous studies [5,11,12]). This approach aims to simulate the quantitative values that are computed in clinical functional brain mapping applications. This makes it possible to test the influence of the optimal spectral band configuration on the quantities measured in clinical applications. For this purpose, the Pearson correlation coefficient is computed. The correlation coefficient was calculated between the theoretical hemodynamic time courses (see Figure 5) and the hemodynamic time courses simulated with the optimal spectral configuration of the hyperspectral camera (see Section 2.6). The correlation coefficient was also computed with the data simulated with RGB imaging. We can also investigate the ability of hyperspectral imaging to monitor the brain metabolism. For this purpose, the Pearson correlation coefficient values were computed between the theoretical oxCCO time course (see Figure 5) and the ΔC_{oxCCO} time courses simulated with the optimal spectral configuration of the hyperspectral camera (see Section 2.6).

We also compared our results with the measurements computed with the gold standard of 121 wavelengths included between 780 nm and 900 nm [23] and with the 8 wavelengths identified by Arifler et al. [27]. For this purpose, we simulated the hemodynamic and/or metabolic monitoring using two or three chromophore systems that used these wavelengths. Note that we did not incorporate noises in these simulations of references.

3. Results

3.1. Determination of the Optimal Spectral Configuration of the Hyperspectral Camera

In Figure 6, the quantification errors in ΔC_{HbO_2}, ΔC_{Hb} and ΔC_{oxCCO} (see Equation (10)) obtained for the best simulation-based deconvolution systems of N spectral bands ($N \in [3; 25]$) are represented. The solid lines stand for the mean quantification error. The colored areas represent the dispersion range of the quantification errors. The vertical dashed lines indicate the optimal number of spectral bands for the deconvolution of each chromophore. Both corrected (in green) and uncorrected spectral configuration (in red) are represented. Note that these data were obtained using noisy measurements; zeros mean Gaussian noises were added to the camera intensities and to the Monte Carlo quantities (mean path length and reflection spectra); see Section 2.6.1.

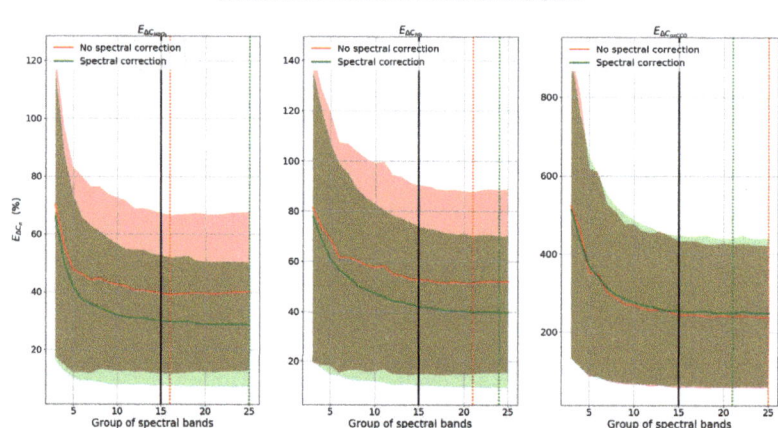

Figure 6. Quantification errors (see Equation (10)) in ΔC_{HbO_2}, ΔC_{Hb}, and ΔC_{oxCCO} obtained for the best simulation-based deconvolution systems of N spectral bands ($N \in [3; 25]$). The solid lines stand for the mean quantification error. The colored areas represent the dispersion range of the quantification errors. The vertical dashed lines indicate the optimal number of spectral bands for the deconvolution of each chromophore. Both corrected (in green) and uncorrected spectral configuration (in red) are represented.

For the three chromophores, the quantification errors are important when a small number of spectral bands are used, but the quantification errors decrease with a larger number of bands. The quantification errors in ΔC_{HbO_2} are on average 30% lower when the spectral correction is applied than when it is not applied. The quantification errors in ΔC_{Hb} are on average 20% lower when the spectral correction is applied than when it is not applied. The quantification errors in ΔC_{oxCCO} are equivalent with and without spectral correction. We can notice that the quantification errors reach a plateau when 15 corrected and uncorrected spectral bands are used. These spectral bands are indicated by violet points in Figure 7 and will be named optimal reduced spectral bands in the rest of the paper.

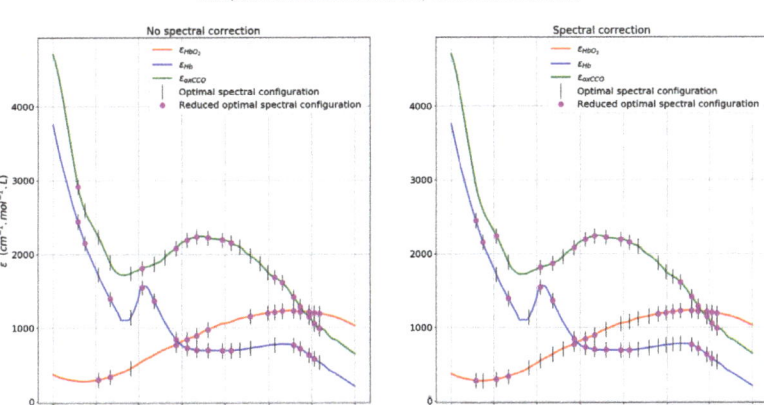

Figure 7. Optimal spectral configuration of the hyperspectral camera XIMEA MQ022HG-IM-SM5X5-NIR obtained with the simulation-based method. The peaks of the selected spectral bands are represented as vertical lines in the molar extinction coefficients of the deconvolved chromophores. The reduced optimal spectral bands are indicated by violet points in the molar extinction coefficients of the deconvolved chromophores.

For each chromophore, different optimal spectral combinations are found. For the quantification of ΔC_{HbO_2}, the best spectral configuration of our hyperspectral camera is composed of 25 spectral bands if the spectral correction is applied and of 16 spectral bands if the spectral correction is not applied. These spectral bands are indicated by black vertical lines in the HbO_2 molar extinction spectra in Figure 7. For these configurations, the quantification error (with Monte Carlo and intensity noise addition) is equal to 28.7% $\pm$ 21.4% (mean $\pm$ standard deviation of the 10^3 measurements) when the spectral correction is applied and is equal to 38.5% $\pm$ 26.9% when the spectral correction is not applied.

For the quantification of ΔC_{Hb}, the best spectral configuration of our hyperspectral camera is composed of 24 spectral bands if the spectral correction is applied and of 21 spectral bands if the spectral correction is not applied. These spectral bands are indicated by black vertical lines in the Hb molar extinction spectra in Figure 7. For these configurations, the quantification error (with Monte Carlo and intensity noise addition) is equal to 39% $\pm$ 29.7% (mean $\pm$ standard deviation of the 10^3 measurements) when the spectral correction is applied and is equal to 49.7% $\pm$ 36.6% when the spectral correction is not applied.

For the quantification of ΔC_{oxCCO}, the best spectral configuration of our hyperspectral camera is composed of 21 spectral bands if the spectral correction is applied and of 25 spectral bands if the spectral correction is not applied. These spectral bands are indicated by black vertical lines in the oxCCO molar extinction spectra in Figure 7. For these configurations, the quantification error (with Monte Carlo and intensity noise addition) is equal to 251.1% $\pm$195.4% (mean $\pm$ standard deviation of the 10^3 measurements) when the spectral correction is applied and is equal to 237.6% $\pm$ 183.1% when the spectral correction is not applied.

Quantification Performances of Deconvolution Systems

When using the optimal or the reduced optimal spectral configurations of the hyperspectral camera (see Figure 7), three linear systems have to be defined to independently quantify ΔC_{HbO_2}, ΔC_{Hb}, and ΔC_{oxCCO}. In the rest of the paper, these systems will be named multiple deconvolution systems. When inspecting the spectral band used in the optimal reduced multiple systems, twenty-one different spectral bands are used with and without spectral correction. Thus, a single system can be designed using these spectral bands to quantify ΔC_{HbO_2}, ΔC_{Hb}, and ΔC_{oxCCO} in a single measurement. In the same way, when inspecting the spectral variables used in the optimal multiple systems, all spectral bands of the hyperspectral camera are used. The accuracy of the quantification of the chromophore n can be measured using the mean and the standard deviation of the quantification error (see Equation (10)). According to ISO 5725-1 standards, the term "accuracy" stands for the trueness of the measurement (mean quantification errors close to 0%) and the repeatability of the measurement (standard deviation of quantification errors close to 0%). The mean and standard deviation values were calculated on 10^3 noisy measurements. These metrics were calculated using the multiple and single deconvolution systems of the hyperspectral camera; see Table 3.

Table 3. Quantification performances of the multiple and single deconvolution systems of the hyperspectral camera.

		Multiple Deconvolution Systems		Single Deconvolution Systems	
		Optimal	Optimal Reduced	Optimal Reduced	All Spectral Bands
Spectral correction	$m(E_{\Delta C_{HbO_2}})$	28.7	29.7	29.1	28.7
	$\sigma(E_{\Delta C_{HbO_2}})$	21.4	23.1	21.9	21.4
	$m(E_{\Delta C_{Hb}})$	39	39.7	39.4	39
	$\sigma(E_{\Delta C_{Hb}})$	29.7	31.1	29.8	29.7
	$m(E_{\Delta C_{oxCCO}})$	251.1	252.1	250.1	250.1
	$\sigma(E_{\Delta C_{oxCCO}})$	195.4	198.9	194	195.2
No spectral correction	$m(E_{\Delta C_{HbO_2}})$	38.5	38.7	40.6	40.6
	$\sigma(E_{\Delta C_{HbO_2}})$	26.9	27.8	28.1	27.3
	$m(E_{\Delta C_{Hb}})$	49.7	50.9	50.5	50.1
	$\sigma(E_{\Delta C_{Hb}})$	36.6	37.5	36.8	36.6
	$m(E_{\Delta C_{oxCCO}})$	237.6	244.3	239.1	237.6
	$\sigma(E_{\Delta C_{oxCCO}})$	183.1	186.5	183.9	183.1

For each chromophore, the lowest values of the mean and standard deviation of the quantification errors in ΔC_{HbO_2} and ΔC_{Hb} are obtained with the optimal multiple deconvolution system using corrected spectral bands. When the spectral bands are not corrected, the mean and standard deviation values of the quantification errors in ΔC_{HbO_2} and ΔC_{Hb} are higher than the values obtained with corrected spectral bands. However, we can notice that the mean and standard deviation values of the quantification errors in ΔC_{oxCCO} computed without spectral correction are lower than the values obtained with corrected spectral bands. The quantification errors computed with the optimal multiple system are similar to those obtained with the single system composed of all the spectral bands of the hyperspectral camera. The quantification errors computed with the optimal reduced multiple system are similar to those obtained with the single optimal reduced system.

3.2. Impact of the Signal-to-Noise Ratio in the Measurements

As mentioned in Section 2.3, the SNR values of the imaging system directly impact the amount of noise and the accuracy of the simulated quantities. To illustrate the effect of SNR on the measurements, the mean and standard deviation of the quantification errors in ΔC_{HbO_2}, ΔC_{Hb} and ΔC_{oxCCO} (see Equation (10)) obtained for the optimal spectral configuration of the hyperspectral camera (see Figure 7) and the RGB camera are represented as a function of SNR; see Figures 8 and 9. For each chromophore system, the mean and standard deviation values of the quantification errors are high for low SNR values and decrease with increasing SNR values.

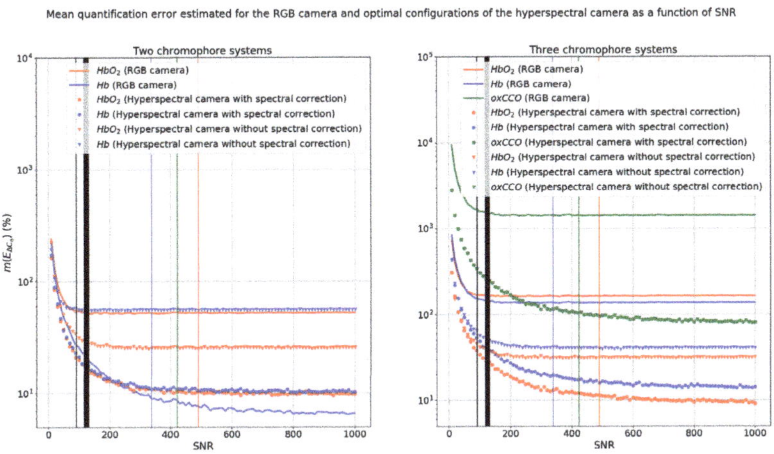

Mean quantification error estimated for the RGB camera and optimal configurations of the hyperspectral camera as a function of SNR

Figure 8. Mean quantification errors in ΔC_{HbO_2} (b), ΔC_{Hb} (blue curves), and ΔC_{oxCCO} (green curves) (see Equation (10)) obtained for the optimal spectral configuration of the hyperspectral camera (see Figure 7) and the RGB camera as a function of SNR. The solid lines were computed using the RGB camera; the curves with circles and with triangles were computed using the hyperspectral camera with and without spectral correction, respectively. Red, green, and blue vertical lines indicate the SNR values of the R, G, and B channels of the RGB camera and black vertical lines the SNR values of the spectral channels of the hyperspectral camera.

Dispersion of the quantification error estimated for the RGB camera and optimal configurations of the hyperspectral camera as a function of SNR

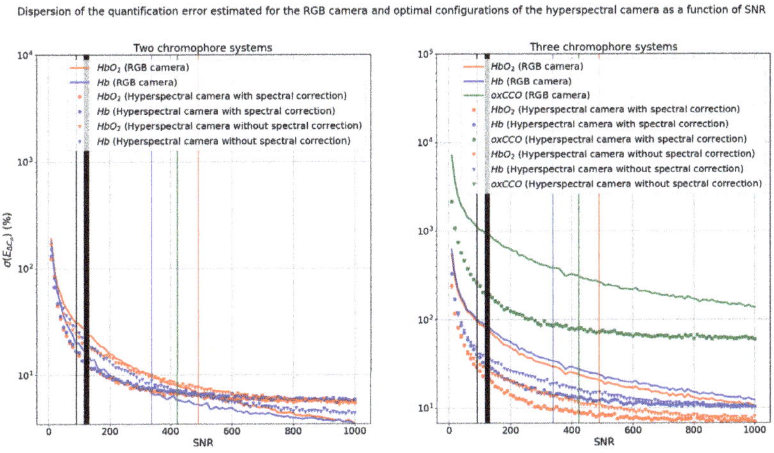

Figure 9. Standard deviation of the quantification errors in ΔC_{HbO_2} (red curves), ΔC_{Hb} (blue curves), and ΔC_{oxCCO} (green curves) (see Equation (10)) obtained for the optimal spectral configuration of the hyperspectral camera (see Figure 7) and the RGB camera as a function of SNR. The solid lines were computed using the RGB camera; the curves with circles and with triangles were computed using the hyperspectral camera with and without spectral correction, respectively. Red, green, and blue vertical lines indicate the SNR values of the R, G, and B channels of the RGB camera and black vertical lines the SNR values of the spectral channels of the hyperspectral camera.

When a two-chromophore system is considered with the RGB camera (SNR = 10), the quantification errors in ΔC_{HbO_2} and ΔC_{Hb} are equal to 236% ± 187% and 226% ± 179%, respectively. When the SNR value is equal to 1000, the quantification errors in ΔC_{HbO_2} and ΔC_{Hb} are equal to 52% ± 3% and 6% ± 3%, respectively. For high SNR values, it is interesting to note that the quantification of ΔC_{HbO_2} is not accurate (low $\sigma(E_{HbO_2})$ values and high $m(E_{HbO_2})$ values) and the quantification of ΔC_{Hb} is accurate. Moreover, the mean quantification errors in ΔC_{HbO_2} reach a plateau for an SNR value equal to 110. For the hyperspectral camera with an SNR value equal to 10, the quantification errors in ΔC_{HbO_2} are equal to 232% ± 173% when the spectral correction is applied and 259% ± 193% when it is not applied. The quantification errors in ΔC_{Hb} are equal to 235% ± 176% when the spectral correction is applied and 267% ± 201% when it is not applied. When the SNR value is equal to 1000, the quantification errors in ΔC_{HbO_2} are equal to 8% ± 6% when the spectral correction is applied and 28% ± 6% when it is not applied. The quantification errors in ΔC_{Hb} are equal to 8% ± 6% when the spectral correction is applied and 52% ± 5% when it is not applied. For high SNR values, the quantification of ΔC_{HbO_2} and ΔC_{Hb} is accurate when the spectral correction is applied and not accurate when the spectral correction is not applied (low $\sigma(E_n)$ values and high $m(E_n)$ values). When the spectral correction is not applied, the mean quantification errors in ΔC_{HbO_2} and ΔC_{Hb} reach a plateau for an SNR value equal to 200 and 110, respectively.

When a three-chromophore system is considered with the RGB camera (SNR = 10), the quantification errors in ΔC_{HbO_2}, ΔC_{Hb}, and ΔC_{oxCCO} are equal to 712% ± 531%, 822% ± 617%, and 9427% ± 7011%, respectively. When the SNR value is equal to 1000, the quantification errors in ΔC_{HbO_2}, ΔC_{Hb}, and ΔC_{oxCCO} are equal to 164% ± 10%, 138% ± 12%, and 1431% ± 138%, respectively. The mean quantification errors in ΔC_{HbO_2}, ΔC_{Hb}, and ΔC_{oxCCO} reach a plateau for an SNR value equal to 110, 130, and 130, respectively. For high SNR values, the quantification of ΔC_{HbO_2}, ΔC_{Hb}, and ΔC_{oxCCO} is not accurate (low $\sigma(E_n)$ values and high $m(E_n)$ values). For the hyperspectral camera with an SNR value equal to 10, the quantification errors in ΔC_{HbO_2} are equal to 345% ± 267% when the spectral correction is applied and 328% ± 248% when it is not applied. The quantification errors in ΔC_{Hb} are equal to 486% ± 379% when the spectral correction is applied and 496% ± 382% when it is not applied. The quantification errors in ΔC_{oxCCO} are equal to 2908% ± 2190% when the spectral correction is applied and 2951% ± 2201% when it is not applied. When the SNR value is equal to 1000, the quantification errors in ΔC_{HbO_2} are equal to 10% ± 8% when the spectral correction is applied and 33% ± 8% when it is not applied. The quantification errors in ΔC_{Hb} are equal to 14% ± 11% when the spectral correction is applied and 41% ± 11% when it is not applied. The quantification errors in ΔC_{oxCCO} are equal to 90% ± 68% when the spectral correction is applied and 91% ± 70% when it is not applied. For high SNR values, the quantification of ΔC_{HbO_2} and ΔC_{Hb} is accurate when the spectral correction is applied and not accurate (low $\sigma(E_n)$ values and high $m(E_n)$ values) when the spectral correction is not applied. The quantification of ΔC_{oxCCO} is not accurate with and without spectral correction (low $\sigma(E_{oxCCO})$ values and high $m(E_{oxCCO})$ values). We can notice that the measurement uncertainty of ΔC_{oxCCO} is similar for all SNR values with and without spectral correction. When the spectral correction is not applied, the mean quantification errors in ΔC_{HbO_2} and ΔC_{Hb} reach a plateau for an SNR value equal to 200.

3.3. Hemodynamic Monitoring

The hemodynamic monitoring (ΔC_{HbO_2} and ΔC_{Hb} measurements) following a simulated patient neuronal stimulation (see Section 2.7) is represented In Figures 10 and 11. In Figure 10, the ΔC_{HbO_2} and ΔC_{Hb} values were computed with the optimal spectral combination of the hyperspectral camera; see Figure 7. In Figure 11, the ΔC_{HbO_2} and ΔC_{Hb} values were computed with the RGB camera. In these figures, the modified Beer–Lambert law was computed 10^3 times, using different Monte Carlo and intensity noise occurrences for each time iteration. When using the 121 wavelengths included between 780 nm and 900 nm [23] to quantify the concentration changes during the stimulation period (from $t = 18$ s to $t = 38$ s), there is a 12% overestimation of the ΔC_{HbO_2} values and a 34% underestimation of the ΔC_{Hb} values compared to the theoretical measurements. When using the eight wavelengths identified by Arifler et al. [27] to quantify the concentration changes during the stimulation period, there is a 13% overestimation of the ΔC_{HbO_2} values and a 31% underestimation of the ΔC_{Hb} values compared to the theoretical measurements.

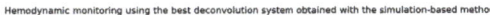
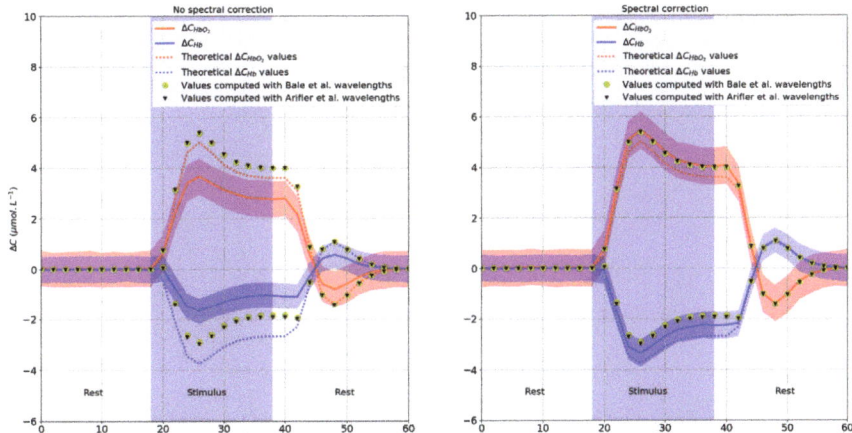

Figure 10. Hemodynamic monitoring following neuronal activation computed with the spectral configuration of the hyperspectral camera obtained with the simulation-based method (see Figure 7). The dashed lines represent the theoretical hemodynamic responses following the neuronal stimulation. The dispersion ranges of the measurements are represented by colored areas. The concentration changes averaged over the 10^3 noisy measurements are represented in solid lines. The concentration changes' time courses computed with the 121 wavelengths included between 780 nm and 900 nm [23] are represented with yellow points. The ones computed with Arifler et al.'s wavelengths [27] are represented with black triangles. The blue rectangle represents the "patient" physiological stimulus.

In Figure 10, the hemodynamic monitoring following a simulated neuronal stimulation was computed using hyperspectral imaging. The optimal corrected and uncorrected spectral configurations of the hyperspectral camera were used to quantify the ΔC_{HbO_2} and ΔC_{Hb} values. The quantification dispersion ranges of the corrected and uncorrected spectral configurations have approximately the same range of magnitude. The standard deviation averaged over all time measurements for ΔC_{HbO_2} and ΔC_{Hb} are equal to 0.9 µmol·L^{-1} and 0.7 µmol·L^{-1}, respectively. When the spectral bands are corrected, the ΔC_{HbO_2} and ΔC_{Hb} values averaged over the 10^3 noisy measurements have a good match with the theoretical hemodynamic responses. During the stimulation period, there is on average a 14% overestimation of the ΔC_{HbO_2} values and a 18% underestimation of the ΔC_{Hb} values compared to the theoretical measurements. When the spectral bands are not corrected, there is on average a 17% underestimation of the ΔC_{HbO_2} values and a 58% underestimation of the ΔC_{Hb} values compared to the theoretical measurements. The correlation coefficients computed between the theoretical HbO$_2$ response and the ΔC_{HbO_2} time courses are higher when the spectral bands are corrected ($r = 0.951 \pm 0.013$) than when they are not ($r = 0.904 \pm 0.026$). In the same way, the correlation coefficients computed between the theoretical Hb response and the ΔC_{Hb} time courses are higher when the spectral bands are corrected ($r = 0.932 \pm 0.018$) than when they are not ($r = 0.783 \pm 0.059$). The correlation coefficient values are summarized in Table 4.

In Figure 11, the hemodynamic monitoring following a simulated neuronal stimulation was computed using RGB imaging. The standard deviation averaged over all time measurements is equal to 0.35 µmol·L^{-1} and 0.20 µmol·L^{-1} for ΔC_{HbO_2} and ΔC_{Hb}, respectively. The ΔC_{HbO_2} values values averaged over the 10^3 noisy measurements do not have a good match with the theoretical HbO$_2$ response; however, the match is rather good between the ΔC_{Hb} values and the theoretical Hb response. During the stimulation period, there is on average a 48% underestimation of the ΔC_{HbO_2} values and a 4% underestimation of the ΔC_{Hb} values compared to the theoretical measurements. The correlation coefficients computed between the theoretical HbO$_2$ response and the ΔC_{HbO_2} time courses are equal to

$r = 0.949 \pm 0.013$. The correlation coefficients computed between the theoretical Hb response and the ΔC_{Hb} time courses are equal to $r = 0.989 \pm 0.002$. The correlation coefficient values are summarized in Table 4.

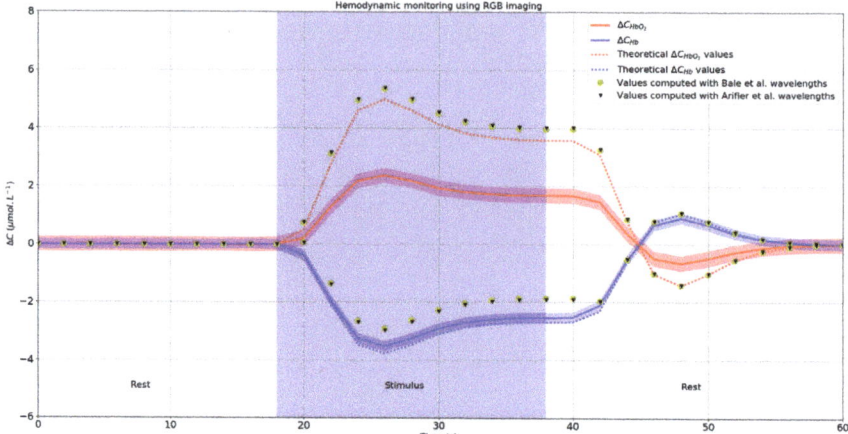

Figure 11. Hemodynamic monitoring following neuronal activation computed with RGB imaging. The dashed lines represent the theoretical hemodynamic responses following the neuronal stimulation. The dispersion ranges of the measurements are represented by colored areas. The concentration changes averaged over the 10^3 noisy measurements are represented in solid lines. The concentration changes' time courses computed with the 121 wavelengths included between 780 nm and 900 nm [23] are represented with yellow points. The ones computed with Arifler et al.'s wavelengths [27] are represented with black triangles. The blue rectangle represents the "patient" physiological stimulus.

Table 4. Pearson correlation coefficients computed between the theoretical hemodynamic responses and the simulated concentration changes' time courses; see Figures 10 and 11. $\mu(r_n)$ and $\sigma(r_n)$ designate the mean and standard deviation, respectively, of the Pearson correlation coefficients computed with the 10^3 noisy time courses of the chromophore n.

	RGB Imaging	Hyperspectral Imaging	
		Spectral Correction	No Spectral Correction
$\mu(r_{HbO_2})$	0.949	0.951	0.904
$\sigma(r_{HbO_2})$	0.013	0.013	0.026
$\mu(r_{Hb})$	0.989	0.932	0.783
$\sigma(r_{Hb})$	0.002	0.018	0.059

3.4. Hemodynamic and Metabolic Monitoring

The hemodynamic and metabolic monitoring (ΔC_{HbO_2}, ΔC_{Hb}, and ΔC_{oxCCO} measurements) following a simulated patient neuronal stimulation (see Section 2.7) are represented in Figures 12 and 13. In Figure 12, the ΔC_{HbO_2}, ΔC_{Hb}, and ΔC_{oxCCO} values were computed with the optimal spectral combination of the hyperspectral camera; see Figure 7. In Figure 13, the ΔC_{HbO_2}, ΔC_{Hb}, and ΔC_{oxCCO} values were computed with the RGB camera. In these figures, the modified Beer–Lambert law was computed 10^3 times, using different Monte Carlo and intensity noise occurrences for each time iteration. When using the 121 wavelengths included between 780 nm and 900 nm [23] to quantify the concentration changes during the stimulation period (from $t = 18$ s to $t = 38$ s), there is a 1.2% underestimation of the ΔC_{HbO_2} values, a 0.4% overestimation of the ΔC_{Hb} values, and a 1.3% overestimation of the ΔC_{oxCCO} values compared to the theoretical measurements.

When using the eight wavelengths identified by Arifler et al. [27] to quantify the concentration changes during the stimulation period, there is a 1.7% underestimation of the ΔC_{HbO_2} values, a 1.91% overestimation of the ΔC_{Hb} values, and a 6% overestimation of the ΔC_{oxCCO} values compared to the theoretical measurements.

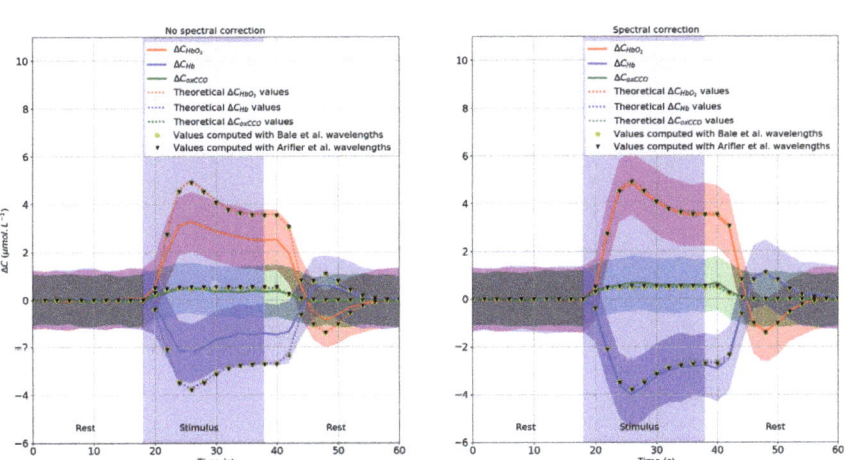

Figure 12. Hemodynamic and metabolic monitoring following neuronal activation computed with the optimal spectral configuration obtained with the simulation-based method (see Figure 7). The dashed lines represent the theoretical hemodynamic and metabolic responses following the neuronal stimulation. The dispersion ranges of the measurements are represented by colored areas. The concentration changes averaged over the 10^3 noisy measurements are represented in solid lines. The concentration changes' time courses computed with the 121 wavelengths included between 780 nm and 900 nm [23] are represented with yellow points. The ones computed with Arifler et al.'s wavelengths [27] are represented with black triangles. The blue rectangle represents the "patient" physiological stimulus.

In Figure 12, the hemodynamic and metabolic monitoring following a simulated neuronal stimulation was computed using hyperspectral imaging. The optimal corrected and uncorrected spectral configurations of the hyperspectral camera were used to quantify the ΔC_{HbO_2}, ΔC_{Hb}, and ΔC_{oxCCO} values. The quantification dispersion ranges of the corrected and uncorrected spectral configurations have approximately the same range of magnitude. The standard deviation averaged over all time measurements for ΔC_{HbO_2}, ΔC_{Hb}, and ΔC_{oxCCO} are equal to 1.23 µmol·L^{-1}, 1.27 µmol·L^{-1}, and 1.07 µmol·L^{-1}, respectively. When the spectral bands are corrected, the ΔC_{HbO_2} and ΔC_{Hb} values averaged over the 10^3 noisy measurements have a good match with the theoretical hemodynamic responses. The ΔC_{oxCCO} values averaged over the 10^3 noisy measurements have a good match with the theoretical metabolic response with and without spectral correction. When the spectral bands are corrected, there is on average a 0.5% underestimation of the ΔC_{HbO_2} values, a 4.4% overestimation of the ΔC_{Hb} values, and a 15% overestimation of the ΔC_{oxCCO} values compared to the theoretical measurements. When the spectral bands are not corrected, there is on average a 25% underestimation of the ΔC_{HbO_2} values, a 42% underestimation of the ΔC_{Hb} values, and a 19% underestimation of the ΔC_{oxCCO} values compared to the theoretical measurements. The correlation coefficients computed between the theoretical HbO$_2$ response and the ΔC_{HbO_2} time courses are higher when the spectral bands are corrected ($r = 0.843 \pm 0.043$) than when they are not ($r = 0.749 \pm 0.068$). The correlation coefficients computed between the theoretical Hb response and the ΔC_{Hb} time courses are higher when the spectral bands are corrected ($r = 0.780 \pm 0.063$) than when they are not ($r = 0.577 \pm 0.112$). The correlation coefficients computed between the theoretical oxCCO response and the ΔC_{oxCCO} time courses are higher when the spectral bands are corrected ($r = 0.256 \pm 0.177$) than when they are not ($r = 0.177 \pm 0.175$). The correlation coefficient values are summarized in Table 5.

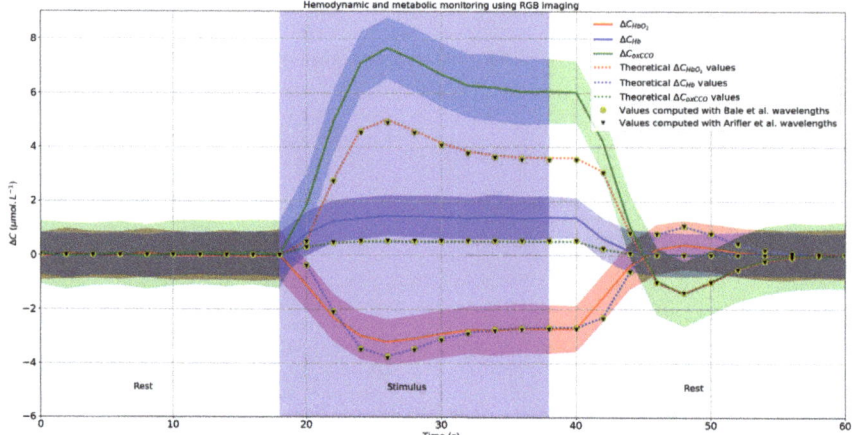

Figure 13. Hemodynamic and metabolic monitoring following neuronal activation computed with RGB imaging. The dashed lines represent the theoretical hemodynamic and metabolic responses following the neuronal stimulation. The dispersion ranges of the measurements are represented by colored areas. The concentration changes averaged over the 10^3 noisy measurements are represented in solid lines. The concentration changes' time courses computed with the 121 wavelengths included between 780 nm and 900 nm [23] are represented with yellow points. The ones computed with Arifler et al.'s wavelengths [27] are represented with black triangles. The blue rectangle represents the "patient" physiological stimulus.

In Figure 13, the hemodynamic and metabolic monitoring following a simulated neuronal stimulation was computed using RGB imaging. The standard deviation averaged over all time measurements is equal to 1.24 µmol·L^{-1}, 1.04 µmol·L^{-1}, and 1.54 µmol·L^{-1} for ΔC_{HbO_2}, ΔC_{Hb}, and ΔC_{oxCCO}, respectively. The computed ΔC_{HbO_2}, ΔC_{Hb}, and ΔC_{oxCCO} values do not have a good match with the theoretical hemodynamic and metabolic responses. During the stimulation period, there is on average a 169% underestimation of the ΔC_{HbO_2} values, a 147% underestimation of the ΔC_{Hb} values, and a 1036% overestimation of the ΔC_{oxCCO} values compared to the theoretical measurements. We can notice that there is an important crosstalk between the chromophores. The ΔC_{HbO_2} values were mainly interpreted as Hb variations, the ΔC_{Hb} values as oxCCO variations, and the ΔC_{oxCCO} as HbO$_2$ variations.

Table 5. Pearson correlation coefficients computed between the theoretical hemodynamic and metabolic responses and the simulated concentration changes' time courses; see Figures 12 and 13. $\mu(r_n)$ and $\sigma(r_n)$ designate the mean and standard deviation, respectively, of the Pearson correlation coefficients computed with the 10^3 noisy time courses of the chromophore n.

	RGB Imaging	Hyperspectral Imaging	
		Spectral Correction	No Spectral Correction
$\mu(r_{HbO_2})$	−0.727	0.843	0.749
$\sigma(r_{HbO_2})$	0.072	0.043	0.068
$\mu(r_{Hb})$	−0.499	0.780	0.577
$\sigma(r_{Hb})$	0.126	0.063	0.112
$\mu(r_{oxCCO})$	0.880	0.256	0.177
$\sigma(r_{oxCCO})$	0.030	0.177	0.175

4. Discussion

Matcher et al. [46] showed that the performance of spectroscopic analysis can be improved by increasing the number of wavelengths of illumination. The results of our study are consistent with Matcher et al.'s results; see Figure 6. The simulation-based method presented in this paper aimed to identify the optimal spectral combination of our hyperspectral camera for the brain hemodynamic and metabolic monitoring. When the spectral bands are corrected, the optimal spectral configuration is composed of 21 and 22 spectral bands; see Figure 7. This configuration could be however reduced from 10 to 12 spectral bands while keeping fairly constant performances. We can observe a plateau in the quantification errors of ΔC_{HbO_2} when 10 or more spectral bands are used. We also can observe a plateau in the quantification errors in ΔC_{Hb} and ΔC_{oxCCO} when 12 or more spectral bands are used; see Figure 6. This reduction of the number of the spectral bands could be interesting for the real-time computation of hemodynamic and metabolic brain maps in the operative room using commercial hyperspectral cameras and for the conception of dedicated cameras used in functional brain mapping studies.

In this study, the optimal spectral configurations were obtained by searching the three chromophores deconvolution systems that minimize the quantification errors in ΔC_{HbO_2}, ΔC_{Hb}, and ΔC_{oxCCO}. Therefore, three different spectral configurations were obtained for the deconvolution of the three chromophores. These spectral configurations, as well as the reference configuration identified by Bale et al. [23] and Arifler et al [27] are represented in Figure 14.

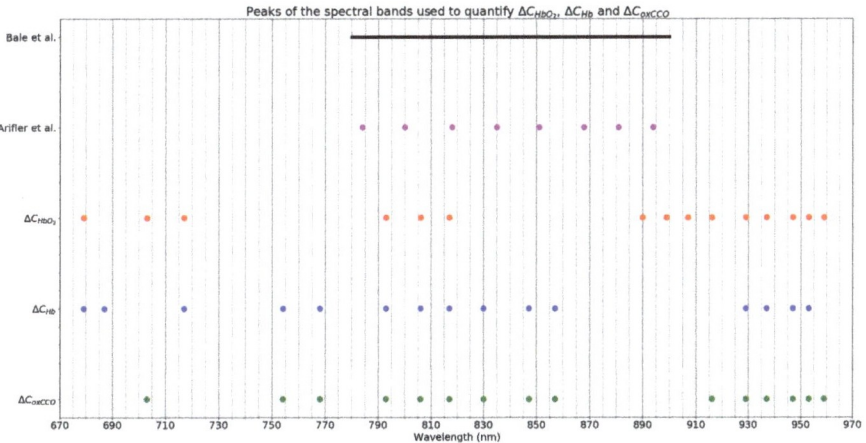

Figure 14. Peaks of spectral bands that minimize the quantification errors in ΔC_{HbO_2}, ΔC_{Hb} and ΔC_{oxCCO}. The spectral configuration identified by Bale et al. [23] and Arifler et al. [27] are also indicated.

The comparison between the spectral configuration identified by Arifler and al. and ours is not trivial since our hyperspectral camera does not acquire exactly the same wavelengths; see Figure 2. There are some similarities between the wavelengths used in our system and in the system of Arifler et al. Indeed, between 780 nm and 900 nm, some wavelengths correspond. Our system also used others wavelengths inferior to 780 nm (703, 754, and 767 nm) and superior to 900 nm (916, 929, 937, 947, 953, and 958 nm). The quantification of ΔC_{HbO_2}, ΔC_{Hb}, and ΔC_{oxCCO} computed with the optimal spectral bands of our hyperspectral camera are consistent with those computed with 121 wavelengths included between 780 nm and 900 nm [23] and with those computed with the eight wavelengths identified by Arifler et al. [27]. For a two-chromophore deconvolution system, the quantification error in ΔC_{HbO_2} measured with our system is equivalent to those measured with 121 wavelengths. However, the choice of our spectral bands aims to reduce the quantification error in ΔC_{Hb}; see Figure 10. For a three-chromophore deconvolution system, the quantification errors measured with our system are a little higher than those measured with 121 wavelengths or with Arifler et al.'s wavelengths; see

Figure 12. This difference may be explained because the illumination and the acquisition of the 121 wavelengths of reference, as well as the eight wavelengths identified by Arifler et al. were simulated as ideal sources and detectors. This means that for these simulations, the term $D \times S$ in Equation (7) is equal to one. To efficiently compare our spectral configuration with these spectral configurations of reference, the spectral sensitivities of the detectors and the illumination sources have to be considered. However, the acquisition condition is different since we acquired the intrinsic signal of an exposed cortex, whereas the wavelengths identified in Bale et al.'s and Arifler et al.'s studies were identified for functional near-infrared spectroscopy devices.

We showed that a spectral correction (see Section 2.2) is required when a hyperspectral mosaic sensor is used [10]. The spectral correction aims to reduce the quantification errors in the measurements and allows a better follows-up of the temporal hemodynamic and metabolic variations; see Table 5.

We also compared hyperspectral imaging to RGB imaging for the computation of hemodynamic and metabolic brain maps. Hyperspectral imaging is the suitable solution to compute hemodynamic maps and metabolic maps thanks to its ability to acquire the intrinsic signal in the near-infrared range [23]. A very important crosstalk between HbO_2, Hb, and oxCCO can be observed when the RGB camera is used for the computation of hemodynamic and metabolic brain maps; see Figure 13. Therefore, RGB imaging is not a suitable solution to compute metabolic brain maps. An RGB camera could be however a low-cost solution to compute hemodynamic maps; see Figure 11. This solution is not accurate to quantify ΔC_{HbO_2}, but is very accurate for the quantification of ΔC_{Hb}. This original result is interesting because most surgical microscopes used in the operating room are equipped with standard RGB cameras. It is known that the BOLD signal used in fMRI studies is predominately due to the paramagnetic properties of deoxygenated hemoglobin [47]. This result indicates that the ΔC_{Hb} quantified with RGB imaging can be used in a robust way for intraoperative functional mapping based on SPM analyses.

We incorporated the camera noises in our simulation to find the most robust and reliable spectral configuration. In Figures 8 and 9, we show that the SNR of the imaging system has a drastic impact on quantification performances. An accurate quantification could be obtained with a high SNR value. Therefore, the light source and the camera specifications and settings have to be carefully chosen in order to guarantee an optimal SNR. This simulation framework could be a great tool for industry or researchers working on intraoperative functional brain mapping solutions to help them in the choice of commercial camera. However, our simulation framework needs to be improved. For the moment, a homogeneous volume of grey matter was considered. A realistic mapping of the exposed cortex could be simulated as suggested by Giannoni et al. [28]. This will be considered in future studies. Moreover, the hemodynamic and metabolic changes following neuronal activation were homogeneously simulated in the volume of grey matter. These events are obviously not consistent with those appearing in a real cortical tissue. This modeling also has to be taken into account to improve our method of identification of the optimal spectral bands of a hyperspectral camera for brain hemodynamic and metabolic monitoring.

5. Conclusions

We present in this paper a method for the identification of the optimal spectral bands of a commercial camera for the intraoperative monitoring of the brain hemodynamic and metabolic responses following neuronal activation. The method described in the report is based on Monte Carlo simulations of the light propagation in a volume of grey matter and incorporates a realistic modeling of the camera acquisition with the addition of Gaussian noises (experimentally measured with the cameras). We identified that an optimal spectral combination of our hyperspectral camera composed of 21 to 22 spectral bands can be used to compute accurate hemodynamic and metabolic brain maps. This configuration could be however reduced from 10 to 12 spectral bands while keeping fairly constant performances, which is consistent with the spectral configurations proposed in the literature. We also showed that RGB imaging is not a suitable technique to compute metabolic brain maps, but is very accurate to compute hemodynamic maps with the quantification of deoxygenated hemoglobin concentration changes. Our Monte Carlo framework needs to be improved, namely with the consideration of the perfusion of grey matter by blood capillaries.

Author Contributions: Conceptualization: C.C., L.M.-W., and B.M. Methodology: C.C., L.M.-W., R.S., M.S., and B.M. Software: C.C., L.M.-W., and M.S. Writing, original draft: C.C. Writing, review and editing: C.C., L.M.-W., R.S., M.S., J.G., and B.M. Supervision: R.S. and B.M. Funding acquisition: R.S. and B.M. Investigation: J.G. Resources: J.G. Project administration: B.M. All authors have read and agreed to the published version of the manuscript.

Funding: These works were funded by LABEX PRIMES (ANR-11-LABX-0063) of Université de Lyon, within the program "Investissements d'Avenir" (ANR-11-IDEX-0007), operated by the French National Research Agency (ANR); Cancéropôle Lyon Auvergne Rhône Alpes (CLARA) within the program "OncoStarter"; Infrastructures d'Avenir en Biologie Santé (ANR-11-INBS-000), within the program "Investissements d'Avenir" operated by the French National Research Agency (ANR) and France Life Imaging.

Acknowledgments: We want to acknowledge the PILoT facility for the support provided for the image acquisition.

Conflicts of Interest: No conflicts of interest, financial or otherwise, are declared by the authors.

Abbreviations

The following abbreviations are used in this manuscript:

HbO_2	Oxygenated hemoglobin
Hb	Deoxygenated hemoglobin
oxCCO	Oxidative state of cytochrome-c-oxidase
BOLD	Blood oxygenation level dependent
fMRI	functional magnetic resonance imaging
NIRS	Near infrared spectroscopy
SPM	Statistical parametric mapping
SNR	Signal-to-noise ratio

References

1. Ogawa, S.; Lee, T.M.; Kay, A.R.; Tank, D.W. Brain magnetic resonance imaging with contrast dependent on blood oxygenation. *Proc. Natl. Acad. Sci. USA* **1990**, *87*, 9868–9872. [CrossRef]
2. Gerard, I.J.; Kersten-Oertel, M.; Petrecca, K.; Sirhan, D.; Hall, J.A.; Collins, D.L. Brain shift in neuronavigation of brain tumors: A review. *Med. Image Anal.* **2017**, *35*, 403–420. [CrossRef] [PubMed]
3. Penfield, W.; Boldrey, E. Somatic motor and sensory representation in the cerebral cortex of man as studied by electrical stimulation. *Brain* **1937**, *60*, 389–443. [CrossRef]
4. Caredda, C.; Mahieu-Williame, L.; Sablong, R.; Sdika, M.; Guyotat, J.; Montcel, B. Real Time Intraoperative Functional Brain Mapping Based on RGB Imaging. *IRBM* **2020**, *1213*, 1–59. [CrossRef]
5. Caredda, C.; Mahieu-Williame, L.; Sablong, R.; Sdika, M.; Alston, L.; Guyotat, J.; Montcel, B. Intraoperative quantitative functional brain mapping using an RGB camera. *Neurophotonics* **2019**, *6*, 1–14. [CrossRef]
6. Karthikeyan, P.; Moradi, S.; Ferdinando, H.; Zhao, Z.; Myllylä, T. Optics Based Label-Free Techniques and Applications in Brain Monitoring. *Appl. Sci.* **2020**, *10*, 2196. [CrossRef]
7. Lu, G.; Fei, B. Medical hyperspectral imaging: A review. *J. Biomed. Opt.* **2014**, *19*, 1–24. [CrossRef]
8. Arridge, S.R.; Cope, M.; Delpy, D.T. The theoretical basis for the determination of optical pathlengths in tissue: temporal and frequency analysis. *Phys. Med. Biol.* **1992**, *37*, 1531–1560. [CrossRef] [PubMed]
9. Kohl-bareis, M.; Ebert, B.; Dreier, J.P.; Leithner, C.; Lindauer, U.; Royl, G. Apparatus for Measuring Blood Parameters. U.S. Patent No. 20120277559, 1 November 2012.
10. Pichette, J.; Laurence, A.; Angulo, L.; Lesage, F.; Bouthillier, A.; Nguyen, D.K.; Leblond, F. Intraoperative video-rate hemodynamic response assessment in human cortex using snapshot hyperspectral optical imaging. *Neurophotonics* **2016**, *3*, 045003. [CrossRef]
11. Caredda, C.; Mahieu-Williame, L.; Sablong, R.; Sdika, M.; Guyotat, J.; Montcel, B. Real time intraoperative functional brain mapping using a RGB camera. In *Clinical and Preclinical Optical Diagnostics II*; Brown, J.Q., van Leeuwen, T.G., Eds.; International Society for Optics and Photonics (SPIE): Washington, DC, USA, 2019; Volume 11073, pp. 17–21. [CrossRef]

12. Caredda, C.; Mahieu-Williame, L.; Sablong, R.; Sdika, M.; Guyotat, J.; Montcel, B. Pixel-wise modified Beer-Lambert model for intraoperative functional brain mapping. In *Clinical and Preclinical Optical Diagnostics II*; Brown, J.Q., van Leeuwen, T.G., Eds.; International Society for Optics and Photonics (SPIE): Washington, DC, USA, 2019; Volume 11073, pp. 148–152. [CrossRef]
13. Hassanpour, M.S.; White, B.R.; Eggebrecht, A.T.; Ferradal, S.L.; Snyder, A.Z.; Culver, J.P. Statistical analysis of high density diffuse optical tomography. *NeuroImage* **2014**, *85*, 104–116. [CrossRef]
14. Ye, J.; Tak, S.; Jang, K.; Jung, J.; Jang, J. NIRS-SPM: Statistical parametric mapping for near-infrared spectroscopy. *NeuroImage* **2009**, *44*, 428–447. [CrossRef] [PubMed]
15. Hillman, E.M.C. Optical brain imaging in vivo: techniques and applications from animal to man. *J. Biomed. Opt.* **2007**, *12*, 051402. [CrossRef] [PubMed]
16. Lange, F.; Peyrin, F.; Montcel, B. Broadband time-resolved multi-channel functional near-infrared spectroscopy system to monitor in vivo physiological changes of human brain activity. *Appl. Opt.* **2018**, *57*, 6417–6429. [CrossRef] [PubMed]
17. Mottin, S.; Montcel, B.; Guillet de Chatellus, H.; Ramstein, S. Functional white laser imaging to study brain oxygen uncoupling/re-coupling in songbirds. *J. Cereb. Blood Flow Metab. Off. J. Int. Soc. Cereb. Blood Flow Metab.* **2010**, *31*, 393–400. [CrossRef]
18. Mottin, S.; Montcel, B.; Chatelus, H.; Ramstein, S.; Vignal, C.; Mathevon, N. CORRIGENDUM: Functional white laser imaging to study brain oxygen uncoupling/re-coupling in songbirds. *J. Cereb. Blood Flow Metab. Off. J. Int. Soc. Cereb. Blood Flow Metab.* **2011**, *31*, 1170. [CrossRef]
19. Vignal, C.; Boumans, T.; Montcel, B.; Ramstein, S.; Verhoye, M.; Van Audekerke, J.; Mathevon, N.; Van Der Linden, A.; Mottin, S. Measuring brain hemodynamic changes in a songbird: Responses to hypercapnia measured with functional MRI and near-infrared spectroscopy. *Phys. Med. Biol.* **2008**, *53*, 2457–2470. [CrossRef]
20. Montcel, B.; Chabrier, R.; Poulet, P. Time-resolved absorption and haemoglobin concentration difference maps: A method to retrieve depth-related information on cerebral hemodynamics. *Opt. Express* **2006**, *14*, 12271–12287. Available online: https://www.osapublishing.org/DirectPDFAccess/D392522C-0D5D-A58B-B00C065E3FE3DED9_119770/oe-14-25-12271.pdf?da=1&id=119770&seq=0&mobile=no (accessed on 1 June 2020). [CrossRef]
21. Montcel, B.; Chabrier, R.; Poulet, P. Detection of cortical activation with time-resolved diffuse optical methods. *Appl. Opt.* **2005**, *44*, 1942–1947. [CrossRef]
22. Wong-Riley, M.T. Cytochrome oxidase: An endogenous metabolic marker for neuronal activity. *Trends Neurosci.* **1989**, *12*, 94–101. [CrossRef]
23. Bale, G.; Elwell, C.E.; Tachtsidis, I. From Jöbsis to the present day: A review of clinical near-infrared spectroscopy measurements of cerebral cytochrome-c-oxidase. *J. Biomed. Opt.* **2016**, *21*, 091307. [CrossRef]
24. Giannoni, L.; Lange, F.; Davies, A.L.; Dua, A.; Gustavson, B.; Smith, K.J.; Tachtsidis, I. Hyperspectral Imaging of the Hemodynamic and Metabolic States of the Exposed Cortex: Investigating a Commercial Snapshot Solution. In *Oxygen Transport to Tissue XL*; Thews, O., LaManna, J.C., Harrison, D.K., Eds.; Springer International Publishing: Cham, Switzerland, 2018; pp. 13–20. [CrossRef]
25. Caredda, C.; Mahieu-Williame, L.; Sablong, R.; Sdika, M.; Guyotat, J.; Montcel, B. Intraoperative functional and metabolic brain mapping using hyperspectral imaging. In *Clinical and Translational Neurophotonics 2020*; Madsen, S.J., Yang, V.X.D., Thakor, N.V., Eds.; International Society for Optics and Photonics (SPIE): Washington, DC, USA, 2020; Volume 11225, pp. 24–30. [CrossRef]
26. Mori, M.; Chiba, T.; Nakamizo, A.; Kumashiro, R.; Murata, M.; Akahoshi, T.; Tomikawa, M.; Kikkawa, Y.; Yoshimoto, K.; Mizoguchi, M.; et al. Intraoperative visualization of cerebral oxygenation using hyperspectral image data: a two-dimensional mapping method. *Int. J. Comput. Assist. Radiol. Surg.* **2014**, *9*, 1059–1072. [CrossRef]
27. Arifler, D.; Zhu, T.; Madaan, S.; Tachtsidis, I. Optimal wavelength combinations for near-infrared spectroscopic monitoring of changes in brain tissue hemoglobin and cytochrome c oxidase concentrations. *Biomed. Opt. Express* **2015**, *6*, 933–947. [CrossRef]
28. Giannoni, L.; Lange, F.; Tachtsidis, I. Investigation of the quantification of hemoglobin and cytochrome-c-oxidase in the exposed cortex with near-infrared hyperspectral imaging: A simulation study. *J. Biomed. Opt.* **2020**, *25*, 1–25. [CrossRef] [PubMed]

29. Sudakou, A.; Wojtkiewicz, S.; Lange, F.; Gerega, A.; Sawosz, P.; Tachtsidis, I.; Liebert, A. Depth-resolved assessment of changes in concentration of chromophores using time-resolved near-infrared spectroscopy: estimation of cytochrome-c-oxidase uncertainty by Monte Carlo simulations. *Biomed. Opt. Express* **2019**, *10*, 4621–4635. [CrossRef]
30. Chen, L.Y.; Pan, M.C.; Yan, C.C.; Pan, M.C. Wavelength optimization using available laser diodes in spectral near-infrared optical tomography. *Appl. Opt.* **2016**, *55*, 5729–5737. [CrossRef] [PubMed]
31. Ocean Optics. USB 2000 Spectrometer. Available online: www.ugastro.berkeley.edu (accessed on 1 June 2020).
32. Bayer, B.E. Color Imaging Array. U.S. Patent No. 3971065 A, 20 July 1976. p. 10.
33. Benoit, L.; Benoit, R.; Belin, E.; Vadaine, R.; Demilly, D.; Chapeau-Blondeau, F.; Rousseau, D. On the value of the Kullback–Leibler divergence for cost-effective spectral imaging of plants by optimal selection of wavebands. *Mach. Vis. Appl.* **2016**, *27*, 625–635. [CrossRef]
34. Fang, Q.; Boas, D.A. Monte Carlo simulation of photon migration in 3D turbid media accelerated by graphics processing units. *Opt. Express* **2009**, *17*, 20178–20190. [CrossRef]
35. Schotland, J.C.; Haselgrove, J.C.; Leigh, J.S. Photon hitting density. *Appl. Opt.* **1993**, *32*, 448–453. [CrossRef] [PubMed]
36. Mitchell, H.H.; Hamilton, T.S.; Steggerda, F.R.; Bean, H.W. The chemical composition of the adult human body and its bearing on the biochemistry of growth. *J. Biol. Chem.* **1945**, *158*, 625–637. Available online: https://www.jbc.org/content/158/3/625.full.pdf (accessed on 1 June 2020).
37. Gagnon, L.; Gauthier, C.; Hoge, R.D.; Lesage, F.; Selb, J.; Boas, D.A. Double-layer estimation of intra- and extracerebral hemoglobin concentration with a time-resolved system. *J. Biomed. Opt.* **2008**, *13*, 054019. [CrossRef]
38. Binding, J.; Ben Arous, J.; Léger, J.F.; Gigan, S.; Boccara, C.; Bourdieu, L. Brain refractive index measured in vivo with high-NA defocus-corrected full-field OCT and consequences for two-photon microscopy. *Opt. Express* **2011**, *19*, 4833. [CrossRef] [PubMed]
39. Jacques, S.L. Optical properties of biological tissues: A review. *Phys. Med. Biol.* **2013**, *58*, R37–R61. [CrossRef] [PubMed]
40. Cope, M. The Application of Near Infrared Spectroscopy to Non Invasive Monitoring of Cerebral Oxygenation in the Newborn Infant. Ph.D. Thesis, University College London, London, UK, 1991.
41. Mason, M.G.; Nicholls, P.; Cooper, C.E. Re-evaluation of the near-infrared spectra of mitochondrial cytochrome c oxidase: Implications for non invasive in vivo monitoring of tissues. *Biochim. Biophys. Acta Bioenerg* **2014**, *1837*, 1882–1891. [CrossRef]
42. Yaroslavsky, A.N.; Schulze, P.C.; Yaroslavsky, I.V.; Schober, R.; Ulrich, F.; Schwarzmaier, H.J. Optical properties of selected native and coagulated human brain tissues in vitro in the visible and near-infrared spectral range. *Phys. Med. Biol.* **2002**, *47*, 2059–2073. [CrossRef] [PubMed]
43. Steimers, A.; Gramer, M.; Ebert, B.; Füchtemeier, M.; Royl, G.; Leithner, C.; Dreier, J.P.; Lindauer, U.; Kohl-Bareis, M. *Imaging of Cortical Haemoglobin Concentration with RGB Reflectometry*; Optical Society of America: Washington, DC, USA, 2009; p. 736813. [CrossRef]
44. Delpy, D.T.; Cope, M.; Zee, P.v.d.; Arridge, S.; Wray, S.; Wyatt, J. Estimation of optical pathlength through tissue from direct time of flight measurement. *Phys. Med. Biol.* **1988**, *33*, 1433–1442. [CrossRef] [PubMed]
45. Wobst, P.; Wenzel, R.; Kohl, M.; Obrig, H.; Villringer, A. Linear Aspects of Changes in Deoxygenated Hemoglobin Concentration and Cytochrome Oxidase Oxidation during Brain Activation. *NeuroImage* **2001**, *13*, 520–530. [CrossRef]
46. Matcher, S.; Elwell, C.; Cooper, C.; Cope, M.; Delpy, D. Performance Comparison of Several Published Tissue Near-Infrared Spectroscopy Algorithms. *Anal. Biochem.* **1995**, *227*, 54–68. [CrossRef] [PubMed]
47. Culver, J.P.; Siegel, A.M.; Franceschini, M.A.; Mandeville, J.B.; Boas, D.A. Evidence that cerebral blood volume can provide brain activation maps with better spatial resolution than deoxygenated hemoglobin. *NeuroImage* **2005**, *27*, 947–959. [CrossRef] [PubMed]

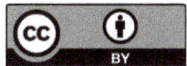

© 2020 by the authors. Licensee MDPI, Basel, Switzerland. This article is an open access article distributed under the terms and conditions of the Creative Commons Attribution (CC BY) license (http://creativecommons.org/licenses/by/4.0/).

MDPI
St. Alban-Anlage 66
4052 Basel
Switzerland
Tel. +41 61 683 77 34
Fax +41 61 302 89 18
www.mdpi.com

Applied Sciences Editorial Office
E-mail: applsci@mdpi.com
www.mdpi.com/journal/applsci

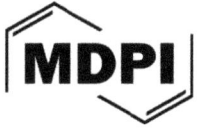

www.ingramcontent.com/pod-product-compliance
Lightning Source LLC
LaVergne TN
LVHW070546100526
838202LV00012B/396